Afternoons with Ivy

Slaying the Dragon of Cancer

3rd Edition

Patti Gray-Pickering

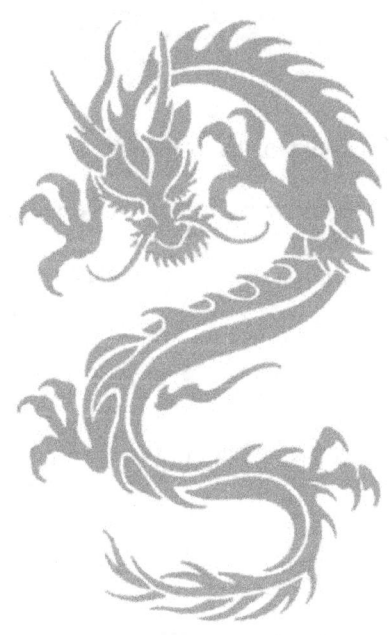

Afternoons with Ivy

Copyright © 2010 by Patti Gray-Pickering

ISBN 1453735879

This book is dedicated to Heidi Goodbar, who lost her battle with her dragon.

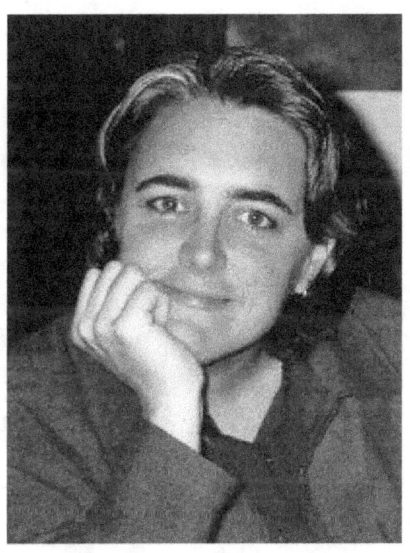

Heidi Lin Goodbar
(December 28, 1970 - July 24, 2006)

Acknowledgments

My heartfelt gratitude goes to all those incredible people that went the extra mile, providing meals, transportation, and prayerful support. You know who you are and I couldn't have done it without you! I love you!

Special thanks to my BFF, Linda, who handled all the details that I couldn't begin to remember, and my husband 'Mas, who provided more comfort than I can ever count. You truly are my soul mate!

Foreword

My right breast lump was discovered around April 1, 2009, but as a tax practitioner, I waited until after tax season to have it checked. I visited my doctor on May 12 and he suspected a malignancy. My digital mammogram was performed on May 13. I was diagnosed with cancer on May 14. I met my surgeon on May 28 and my biopsy was performed on June 4 when a 3.6cm (golf ball sized) malignant tumor was removed. A frozen section and sentinel node dissection were also performed. Since 3 out of 4 nodes showed metastatic carcinoma, six more axillary nodes were removed, one of which had metastatic carcinoma. I met with my oncologist for the first time June 12 and again on June 23. A medi-port was surgically inserted on June 29 and chemotherapy was scheduled to start on June 30. I will testify from personal experience that invasive cancer CAN hurt.

I have infiltrating ductal adenocarcinoma, T2N2Mx, Stage IIIC, as well as ductal carcinoma insitu. I will be undergoing chemotherapy with a TC cocktail (taxotere & cytoxin) through a medi-port once every 3 weeks for up to 6 treatments, at which time I will be facing at least one mastectomy, radiation, and breast reconstruction. My prognostic markers are positive and my HER2 is barely negative.

Update- as of 10/30/2009, cancer has been discovered bilaterally in both lungs. Radiation and mastectomy is canceled. There is no cure.

Table of Contents

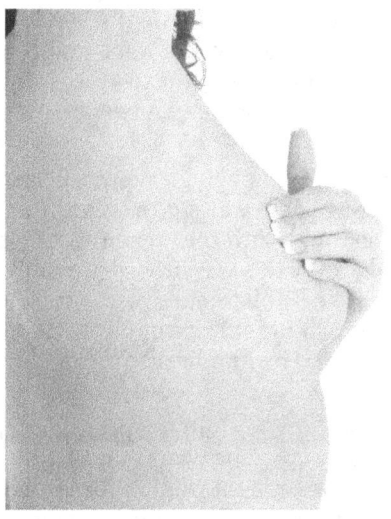

Photo by Kevin Browne

Today was my biopsy. In one sense I am afraid, yet, I am glad to be finding out something more concrete instead of all this speculation. How did I get to this point? They say hindsight is always 20/20, and I am ever the analyst.

I was in the midst of tax season when I first noticed the lump. Actually, it wasn't the lump I noticed but rather the discomfort that the lump generated. It was strong enough to grab my attention. In hindsight I ask myself why I didn't do something right then and there. I'm a tax practitioner and the April 15th deadline was looming. Running three businesses kept me hopping, and at my age, hopping isn't as simple as it used to be! I have always had fibroid breast disease, so lumps and soreness weren't entirely new. I had long since stopped performing self exams, since little lumps were common, and although they would send me jumping through hoops, they never developed into anything. In my mind, this was probably just more of the same. Surely it could wait until after tax season ended.

I was surprised to discover that along with the pain was a sizeable lump in my right breast, almost to the armpit. I pondered how something that size could appear without my knowledge and committed to visiting the doctor after my tax season ended.

During the weeks that followed, the soreness would never completely dissipate, but would wane to varying levels of discomfort. Everything from "don't touch" to "don't breathe" around it. Just when I thought I should run to the doctor for a checkup, the pain would wane and become tolerable, and I would think to myself that it must be going away, satisfying myself that this discomfort was merely a repeat of pains I had experienced in the past.

Finally, early in May, I decided that being safe was better than being sorry. I would put this off no longer. There was a growing concern gnawing in my gut that something was very wrong. With the encouragement of friends, I had convinced myself that whatever this was, it was probably going to be a mere inconvenience and nothing to be over reactive about. It had gotten larger, and could be seen just beneath the surface of my skin as a golf ball size bulge. It was hard. Was it supposed to be that hard?

I sat in the doctor's office waiting for him to appear and tell me that my fears were groundless. "Just a fatty cyst," he would say. "They are always benign". But that isn't what he said. He thought it might be malignant. Malignant?? There is an onus to that word. Everyone knows what malignant means. Did he just say malignant? Suddenly I wished that I had brought my husband with me to this appointment. Next step, a mammogram. Let's not rush to judgment! A mammogram will tell the tale. Ah, a sliver of hope. Now my denial can kick in. The mammogram will prove him wrong and make everything better. A kiss for my boo-boo. The test was scheduled for 8 a.m. "Why so early?" I asked. The pathologist is present to read the x-ray right away at 8 a.m. Between the lines I read, "we want these films read immediately. No waiting." This is turning into a bad horror flick.

Read it, he did. I was told that I would have the results in a couple of days. What a long two days that became. The radiologist's lips were sealed tightly. I watched as she marked various points on the films, wondering what in the world she could see. I saw nothing but black spaces. The mashing process of a mammogram was uncomfortable considering the lump was already sore. But mash she did, again and again. Are we done yet??

Two days later I found a message on my answering machine. The doctor himself. Wow! Usually you get the voice of the nurse. That can't be good. I returned the call, and once again was surprised that I didn't get his nurse. The person on the other end fetched the doctor to the phone. He calmly and politely announced that the mammogram revealed a "lump suspicious of malignancy". I was given options for biopsy and choices of surgeons. Even though my mother had developed post-menopausal cancer some years ago, I had been misinformed that post-menopausal cancer is not genetic, so I blew it off. Cancer wasn't even on my radar! Now her cancer was back on the table and I was devoid of knowledge to this elusive dragon that was lurking behind me. I must Google! With the promise to get back to my doctor with a decision the following Monday, I velcroed myself to my keyboard and began to search.

As I readied myself for bed that night, I stood in front of the mirror in shock. The whole side of my breast was concave! I felt the panic hit me in waves. This wasn't present before the mammogram. The dimple that I had always coveted as a child for my cheek had now found its place in the side of my breast! Dimple is a very apt word for what it looks like.

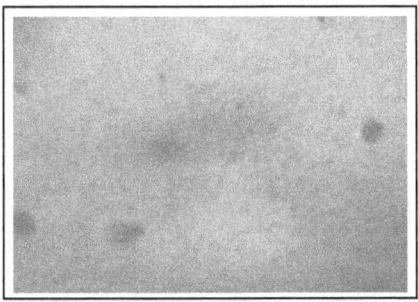

My choices actually were settled within 24 hours so the weekend of pondering was not required. The next step was a consultation with my surgeon of choice. This time I took a backup, and my husband accompanied me to the surgeon's office. I arrived armed with a list of 20 questions, all of which the doctor patiently answered. When he first positioned himself on his little wheeled stool, he announced that if he were a betting man, he would put money on my lump being malignant. Since this had been what I was hearing from the get-go, his confidence didn't come as a surprise to me. The same could not be said of my spouse. The pain had also changed by then to a burning and stinging sensation. The surgeon explained that the tumor was growing and pushing against my breast tissues.

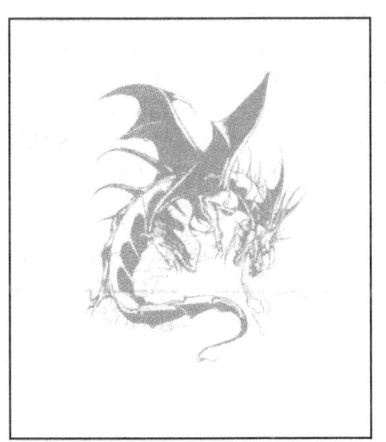

The word "lump" has an innocence to it that doesn't seem so threatening. Suddenly my "lump" became a fire breathing dragon and I wanted it dead! "Out, out damn spot!" The plans for the open biopsy and frozen section were solidified and we silently left the surgeon's office. We left with a plan, but the plan was bereft with an overwhelming sense of dread. My husband cried for the next 24 hours. It broke my heart to see him struggling like a dying man gasping for breath, but I was powerless to fix it. (Did I mention that I'm a fixer?) I considered putting on a plastic smile and

3

dancing my best jig in the hopes of lifting his burden, but I knew that I was about to undertake a difficult process, and I would never be able to maintain such a facade.

The days prior to the biopsy were likened to a roller coaster thrill ride, revealing a new emotion around every turn. By the time the biopsy day arrived, we were anxious to put a face on this dragon and begin the arduous task of slaying it. I did everything I was told to do. No food, no water... which was not that difficult since my appetite had sunk to the depths with my enthusiasm, with one exception...as I backed the car out of the driveway, I popped a piece of nicotine gum into my mouth to arrest my jangled nerves.

I must give the hospital credit due. They processed me in quickly, and I was greeted by a friendly, smiling nurse which seemed a welcome sight amidst all this strangeness. Ushered into my sterile cubicle, I now faced an old, but familiar adversary in the form of a needle. I've always hated needles. When God passed out the masochistic genes he skipped me completely. I put on my brave face, focused on my husband's eyes, breathed deeply, and endured. As usual, my veins had a different agenda than I did and resisted that needle but our team finally scored the touchdown and the needle slipped into its new home in my arm.

As a diabetic, I required a sugar reading that was too high. I had come too far for this obstacle to slow me down. A bit of insulin would resolve the problem. A visit from an aloof anesthesiologist took us to the next level of our journey. "Is that gum in your mouth?" she asked disapprovingly. Little did I know, (they didn't say I couldn't chew gum!) that this little piece of gum would cause so much trouble! As it turned out, the gum produces saliva, which affects the stomach acids, and creates a risk of aspiration. There's another malicious word that I recognized, since my mother had died as a result of aspirating three months earlier. It's amazing how much we attribute to certain words! Malignant, aspirate...words loaded with dynamite just looking for a place to explode. Now, a four hour window was needed to overcome this obstacle, by which time the pathologist and the frozen section would be unavailable. The frozen section represented answers that we very much needed to hear, and losing that possibility was unacceptable. No, I am not interested in rescheduling. I endured that needle, I'm here expecting answers before I leave this day, and in my mind it was "Forward Ho!". After waiving any hospital liability in the event I died from aspirating, we were finally in motion again!

Why are surgical suites so darned cold? I understand that bacteria are minimized in cold environments, but does it have to be SO cold?? Praise God for heated blankets! I prayed that God would let the drugs knock me out quickly. All that talk of putting a tube down my throat scared me to death. I had only had anesthesia one other time in my life, and that was too long ago for my aging memory to conjure up. Why is the unknown so scary? My courage seems to have locked itself in the bathroom, leaving me to fend for myself. Blessedly, sleep came quickly and deeply and I awoke back in my cubicle to my husband's familiar touch. Next best thing to a security blanket in my book!

I was actually awake when my surgeon came to call, but there is little of what he said to me that I remember clearly. A few phrases stuck. My cancer was "malignant" and "on the move". I wondered what the latter meant, but didn't ask. I think I didn't really want to know at that point, although in hindsight, I wish I had asked. Luckily, my husband's antennae were alert, and he caught every word so that he could explain it to me later. Somebody mentioned "no clean margins" and "cancerous sentinel node". I learned that the rest of my accessible lymph nodes had been removed. We had decided at the get-go that a mastectomy would not be performed at this time so I knew that my body was still intact as I knew it to be before the surgery. There was some comfort in that! So much of what was happening to me was unfamiliar, that a bit of familiarity was welcome.

It was suggested that I spend the night in the hospital instead of going home. My head was reeling with everything I was being told. That dragon was breathing fire on the back of my neck and my knees were knocking fiercely! I mentally jotted a list of what-ifs that destabilized the security of home. What if I started bleeding too much? What if I fell? What if, what if, what if...lots of irrational what ifs. My brain kept telling me to get over myself, but the rest of me quaked in my boots! I finally decided to stay in the hospital for the night. There was a safe sense in the knowledge that qualified personnel would only be a click away in the event that any or all of my what-if monsters actually crawled out from beneath the bed. With the light of day, as typically happens, the monsters beneath my bed disappeared and home became the very place that I wanted to be.

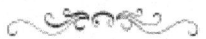

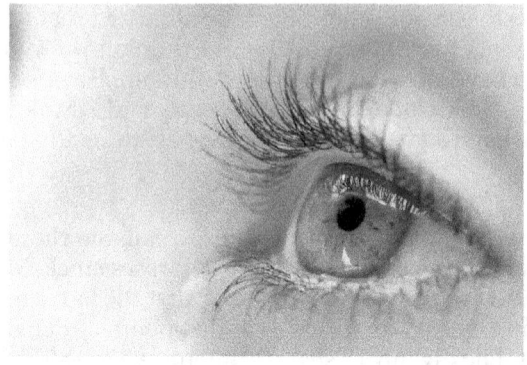

Photo by Enrique Ramos López

What Cancer Cannot Do

It cannot cripple love or shatter hope

It cannot corrode faith or destroy peace

It cannot kill friendship or suppress memories

It cannot silence courage or invade the soul

It cannot steal eternal life or conquer the Spirit

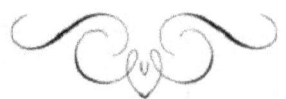

Cancer: The Pathology-Tuesday, June 9, 2009

I've never been much of a people watcher, but as I situated myself in the doctor's waiting room, I found myself scanning the faces of the others present wondering why they were there. Are any of these people waiting for news like I am? Do any of these folks have cancer too? They all seemed calm to me. Do I appear calm to them? Can they see the churning going on in my stomach? Can they see the fear in my eyes? One woman smiled across the room at me. Did I smile back? Does it matter if I didn't?

The wait wasn't long. Why can't getting in and getting out be this easy when you have a hang nail? When the doctor entered the room he explained that the pathologist hadn't finished the written version of the report yet, so I was going to get the paraphrased version. Figures! "The dude has only had 5 days and a staff of how many to assemble on paper what he already knows about what he saw on Thursday" was made a statement by the rolling of my eyes. I made it known that I wanted, no, EXPECTED a copy of that report as fast as the surgeon received it. No snail mails...FAX it! Should I be so pushy? I pondered that for...15 seconds and decided that yes, I was entitled. I figured that now was the time to rehearse my speech about my intention to stay actively involved in this whole process and he may as well be the first to be anointed. I like this surgeon, so saying it nice was pretty easy this time around.

First order of business was to remove the drain tube. "Will this hurt?" I asked. Something about yanking a long piece of plastic that was sewn into my body is intimidating to me. His response was, "hardly". I advised him that "hardly" was the wrong answer. I was looking for a definitive NO. Truth was, I didn't feel it slide out at all, so I sighed a grateful sigh of relief and braced myself for what was coming next. He announced that we needed to talk. Ya think? I curled my fingernails into the soft foam of the table I was perched upon and waited, wondering if the words he spoke would hold any surprises. They didn't much.

He recapped that the tumor didn't contain any clean margins. I knew that already. I didn't know that they went back more than once in an effort to locate some clean margins and finally dug all the way to the muscle of my chest wall before they found any. Boy am I glad I was asleep! No wonder my shoulder blade hurts! The sentinel node was cancerous so removing as many as they could translated into a total of 10. No wonder my arm feels the size of an elephant's leg! I felt better about skipping the needle biopsy in lieu of the lumpectomy right at the get-go. The good news of this visit can be summed up in a mere sentence: Of the 10 nodes removed, only 4 were cancer riddled.

Afternoons with Ivy

Not a very big sentence is it? At least it didn't seem so at the time. Of all the words spoken in that room last night, only ten of them were actually encouraging. I have since decided that this sentence is actually a very BIG sentence because it may well define the difference between living and dying for me. But, more about that later.

So Doc, tell me something I didn't know. He did. The cancer was *very* aggressive. "High Grade" he called it. I know I have the memory of a gnat, but I had to have 'Mas repeat that phrase to me several times before I managed to retain it. When they first spotted the cancer it was already 3.3cm which was large by most standards. By the time they got it out a week later, it was actually 3.6cm. I knew that it was growing because I could feel it, so it was no surprise that it hurt.

He also advised me that I had a second form of cancer permeating my breast tissue. They call it DCIS cancer and it is a slow growing form which is very treatable with radiation. There was too much of that to remove without a mastectomy which may come later, but no matter, because if radiation can kill it, chemotherapy will act like an atom bomb to it, thus making it a back burner issue. The focus is definitely the "high grade" cancer that found it's way to those 4 lymph nodes and is probably currently luxuriating on a cruise through the river of blood inside my body, with ports of call at various places along the route.

Without benefit of a written report, my next question pertains to staging which I know is afforded along with the paper version of the pathology results. Not really news here either. They stop just short of pronouncing this to be a stage 4 because they aren't sure how much of the cancer is on that cruise, and where the ports of call are located. Hmmm, is that glass half full or half empty? Because of the aggressive growth of the cancer, they are assuming the worst, so they intend to attack it with vigor through chemotherapy. Although the outside of my surgical wound is healing nicely, the surgeon indicated that they trashed the inside in search of those clean margins, so there remains some healing to be done. I can't help but notice the snicker curling the lips of that dragon as she leans over my shoulder and puffs a bit of smoke just to remind me of her presence. Damn dragon. I once heard Johnny Carson utter a curse that I thought was worth remembering: May the fleas of a thousand camels infest your armpits. I wonder if dragons can get fleas.

We left the office with the understanding that I would get a call from an oncologist. I got that this morning. Who is this guy? Where did he graduate in his class? Interestingly, your class standing is the LAST thing on your mind when you graduate. I graduated 16 in a class of 200+

and at that time it was much less important to me than driving through Hardee's to grab a coke. Suddenly, the standard takes on new meaning! If I knew then what I know now, would it have....NAH, probably not! Would it be less than PC to ask this guy, "how many were in your graduating class and where did you fit among those numbers? Top or bottom? Were you an honor student or a slacker?"

We walked to the car assembling what we each had heard from our visit. That was an interesting chat. 'Mas, as the powerless spouse prowling through the words for whatever positive he could grasp zeroed in on the 4 out of 10 sentence. I, on the other hand, remembered the "how many Polish people does it take to screw in a light bulb joke, and focused on the knowledge that whether the cancer finds its way to whereabouts unknown through one lymph node or 60 is pretty insignificant if it ultimately gets there at all. Try saying THAT one without any R's. A new challenge was now afoot. When two people, both deeply invested and with very different perspectives are given bad news at the same time, who goes first? Sounds like an Abbot and Costello routine doesn't it? We found ourselves at odds, with 'Mas struggling to maintain a positive focus, and I believing that his unwillingness to examine my viewpoint meant he must certainly be in denial. 'Mas and I are both very passionate people, so disagreements are always interesting at our house. I threw the trump card, "I'm the one who might die!" Bad Patti. It took us 8 blocks of arguing to reach the understanding that we were both right. Hey God, do you wear a black and white striped shirt at these events? Are we allowed to kick dirt on each other? That trump card was definitely dirty.

I thought it was interesting that my husband, who hates to mow grass, perched himself on the John Deere without even coming in the house once the car had been safely nestled in the garage. I'm figuring he needed some alone time, which may signal bad news for the crabgrass! Our life may be a mess for awhile, but we'll have the best looking lawn in town! We always laugh about the pressure we feel when one of the neighbors mow the lawn next to us. Maybe 'Mas will be applying the pressure for awhile! That's okay. He needs to find places to vent, and the John Deere is new, so I figure it can take it.

Back to those sentences...

I have to reflect on the significance of sentences. We use them all the time for a variety of reasons, sometimes good, often bad. How much power there is in 10 words! "I don't like you," is only four words, but equally powerful. I've always been good at engaging the mouth before developing the words. Note to self: Work on that! I mused about my statement that I was the one dying and wince even now at the effect that must have had on 'Mas. It did silence the argument at that moment, but me thinks that you can win the battle only to lose the war. What a selfish sentence. In the world that I grew up in, I was taught that it was never okay to be about me. Now I find myself wondering if it is okay now. Part of me replays my childhood tapes and thinks the answer is NO. Another part of me recognizes that I need to be at least somewhat selfish so that I can resist the urge to fix this to everyone else's comfort level so that I can channel the necessary energy into slaying my dragon. I'm thinking this would make a good high school debate topic.

I've seen a t-shirt that says, "God, keep your arm around my shoulder and your hand over my mouth". I was tempted to buy it then. Maybe I should reconsider it now. If God does wear a striped ump shirt on occasion, he was probably yelling "foul" when I tossed out that cavalier statement about my untimely demise. Lucky for me I have a best friend who has also worn the "spouse" hat. She has already rapped my knuckles nun style at least twice for that twisted black humor that I can spit out so easily when I am struggling with my demons. She would have really clobbered me last night! I can't take those words back, as much as I would like to, any more than the surgeon can take back the "high grade cancer". Devastating words either way, permanent words too.

It occurs to me that there are really two of us dying right now. Two of us are grieving. My grief and death are no less an issue than 'Mas'. At least if I actually die, I get warm fuzzies from a good place. 'Mas won't have the benefit of those. The potential death of "us" is a death for him too. Maybe I could invent some kind of shock collar, like they make for dogs, so that every time my emotions take the lead and I invoke that caustic repartee, a thousand volts would knock me on my ass. I don't have much time to learn this lesson quickly. I'll settle for a V8 commercial, where I say something moronic, and one of you slaps me in the forehead. Less painful, but probably no less effective.

The fact remains that with the sentence, "10 nodes taken, only 4 cancerous", God has opened a window. I would have preferred a sliding glass patio door, but I'll take what I can get. There is my motivator that I have been seeking. There is the faint light at the end of the tunnel that can send that damn dragon packing. She shadows me, wondering if I saw it. Yeah, I saw it. I'm just a little slow on the uptake. I'm rolling up my sleeves now, as I prepare to kick some scaly butt. The survivor instinct is starting to kick in. It's about time! Where have you been?? 10 minus 4=I can still beat this. It's not much, but I think it is enough. Maybe I should chug some of that nasty raw egg like the athletes do. Uh, no.

I won't say that I am where I need to be yet, but God opened the door a crack, and I have stuck my foot into it. Is that the Rocky theme song I'm hearing? CRANK IT UP! Eye of the tiger! All because of a 10 word sentence. Now where did I hang that superwoman suit?

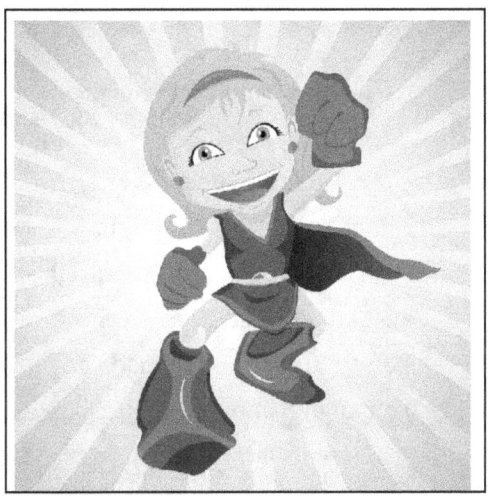

photo by Augusto Cabral

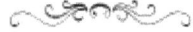

"*Cancer is not a death sentence, but rather it is a life sentence; it pushes one to live.*" ~ *Marcia Smith*

"Stand"

by Rascal Flatts

You feel like a candle in a hurricane
Just like a picture with a broken frame
Alone and helpless
Like you've lost your fight
But you'll be alright, you'll be alright
Cause when push comes to shove
You taste what you're made of
You might bend, till you break
Cause its all you can take
On your knees you look up
Decide you've had enough
You get mad you get strong
Wipe your hands shake it off
Then you Stand, Then you stand
Life's like a novel
With the end ripped out
The edge of a canyon
With only one way down
Take what you're given before its gone
Start holding on, keep holding on
very time you get up
And get back in the race
One more small piece of you
Starts to fall into place

Cancer: It's Thursday!- Thursday, June 11, 2009

I think I'm going to start avoiding Thursdays. Last Thursday was the biopsy that brought bad news. Today is the pathology report that confirms bad news. Maybe I will just strike Thursdays from my calendar.

The fax came a little while ago from the Pathology lab. All SIX pages of it. Too bad I didn't take Greek as a foreign language in high school because then I might have understood a little of it! The explanations contained in the report could fill a "D" cup a lot faster than I can! So many large words! My vocabulary has always been pretty good, but my Google is really getting a workout today! Is there a doctor in the house?? Resorting to my trusty breastcancer.org website I click on the link for deciphering a pathology report and grab my pencil. Let's cut to the chase: Staging. Sounds like a rocket ship getting ready to launch. I wonder why they picked that word to represent the seriousness of a person's cancer? Maybe because you "launch" after you read the report? The letters scattered across the pages are mind numbing. This is the sort of report that I would skip reading at all under normal circumstances. But these aren't normal circumstances, are they? One word in particular leaps off the page: metastasis.

There's that dragon again, nudging me from the rear. Sneering as she flips her tail menacingly. She singed my hair with that one. She swung and she scored. There's something about those M words. malignant, metastasis...no more M words on Thursdays. I feel the hairs begin to tickle the back of my neck. Suddenly my stomach ties itself into knots and I feel sick. I'm frozen to my chair, as though the slightest movement on my part will shatter the air around me, and the space I'm in will crumble like shards of razor sharp glass onto the floor, broken and jagged. Breathe, Patti, breathe!

Yes, metastasis is definitely the gripping word. I already knew that I was a grade 3, I already knew that the cancer was in my lymph nodes, although the odds shifted. Yesterday it was 4 out of 12, now I am 4 out of 10. My percentages have dropped significantly. It's that word metastasis that has me mesmerized. My eyes read it once, twice, and stop there. I'm staring at the page but the page has become a blur. The tears filling my eyes blind me. When does this bad news stop coming?

I read the phrase "infiltrating ductal adenocarcinoma". I don't know anything about that phrase, but it looks important. I cut and paste it into my Google search engine. Histologic type: Infiltrating ductal and lobular carcinomas have the worse prognosis..." My dragon is squeezing me around my chest forcing my breath into shallow wisps of air. Her scaly skin is touching mine and it makes me shudder.

My courage has locked itself in the john again. Some friend that is! Mercifully, 'Mas comes home armed with five very funny cards, a big heart and a large shoulder. Not a minute too soon! I feel as though I take one step forward and two back. Like a suitcase bulging at the seams, I feel as though one more word, one more negative report will split the zipper and send everything toppling to the floor in a jumbled mess!

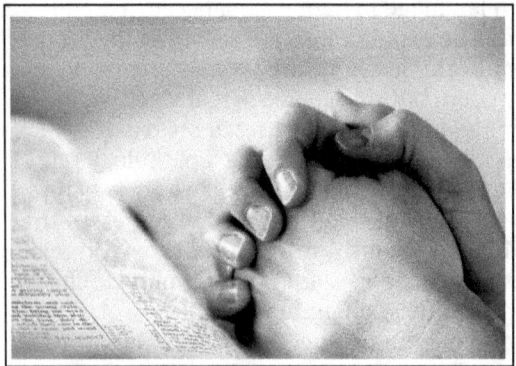

But wait, this is *already* a mess! I call my brother for help understanding this six page jumble of words and numbers. He works in radiology and has always been able to interpret medical mumbo-jumbo for me. He confirms that I "get the gist" and the gist ain't good. He can't make it go away. No one can make it go away. I can't remember ever being this afraid. There must be an "end game" button here somewhere. Am I breathing yet?

It's just too overwhelming...I don't know what to say. I feel myself drawing inward into a fetal position. I don't feel brave today. I don't feel confident today. Today I am not sure that I will live much longer. I mustn't say that out loud though...no one will understand. Everyone will tell me to "buck up" and "think positive". I don't want to today. Because it is Thursday...and nothing good happens on Thursday anymore.

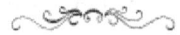

Cancer: The Bigger Picture- Sunday, June 14, 2009

They say there are no atheists in foxholes. Certainly there aren't any in mine. By the end of the week my batteries are pretty tapped out, and I am in need of a recharge. It's a good thing Sunday is coming.

We arrived at church early today because 'Mas had something special he needed to do during the service that left me alone in the pew. As I sat there watching folks come and go, busy doing their thing, it occurred to me that facing mortality forces us to look at life's bigger picture. As I glance up at the big cross that hangs on the alter, I'm comforted knowing that there is more to life than just living to die. It's good to know that at the end of life, there is more than a bleak dark nothingness. It would seem sort of pointless to traverse this journey of life if it held no more meaning than that. THE END. Like watching an gripping movie that ends as the screen suddenly goes dark. No credits. No list of actors. No gracious platitudes. Just a blank, black screen.

and that here is not the last word for me. The world is bigger than me, my cancer is bigger than me, and even though I don't know how this movie is going to end, someone else does. I think that I like the idea that someone else is in control. It's too big a job for me. God knows how my movie is going to end, and whenever that happens, the screen isn't going to abruptly darken. There is going to be more. There is going to be a long list of credits scrolling with the names of all the wonderful friends and family that have contributed so generously from their hearts. The names of people who have impacted my life will go on and on and when that list finally does stop, instead of darkness, the screen will explode with light and music.

I'm not much of a crier. At least I didn't use to be! Lately I can dissolve on a dime. Most often that happens on Sundays, when the worship touches my heart and the powerful presence of God's faithfulness overwhelms me. It is then that I know that no matter how my story ends, I am going to be alright. It's a win-win. If I slay this dragon, I win. If I am unsuccessful, ultimately, I still win. Today was one of those days. As the lyrics appeared on the power point screen, I suddenly found myself on my feet, arms thrust wide open, completely in tune with the message that the song conveys. "Here I am, Lord, send me..."

When we reached the verse-

"When setbacks and failures and upset plans, test my faith and leave me with empty hands, Are You not the closest when it's hardest to stand? I know that You will finish what You began," I began to weep uncontrollably. Not because I was sad. I wept because I was totally overwhelmed by the presence of God, and when God holds you that tightly, you just weep. It's not the first time I've experienced such intensity. The pastor pointed out that faith is a verb rather than a noun, and certainly this must be true. I didn't trust until I met Christ, and since that day (thank you Joy), learning to trust God has been a process, wrought with ups and downs, successes and failures. At times I bend, like a graceful willow in a summer's breeze, but other times I stiffen like an unyielding oak. I felt the comforting shoulders of a friend envelope me while my body shook with sobs. How I would ever trudge through this dark time without the assurance that God is in control and in pace with each step I take is beyond my comprehension.

Koinonia is a Greek word for the special relationship of friends. Old friends started this journey with me many years ago, they are joined by new friends and walk beside me now, and at the end of my story, the faces of friends I haven't seen for a long time will welcome me home. I'm grateful for friends. I know that without the hard work of faith, I would not know the powerful intensity that I am experiencing now. Everything that I have experienced in my life up to this point was somehow meant to be a contribution to the end of my story.

This isn't intended to be a "poor me" post. It's intended to be a grateful and humble acknowledgement of the restoration that God has blessed me with, the people that he has used to accomplish the task, and the security He has given me that my movie doesn't end with a blank, black screen. In the end, I cannot ask for better than that. At such time that you view my movie, remember that it has a happy ending, because where there is God, there is always hope. It's a bigger picture. Lights, camera, action...

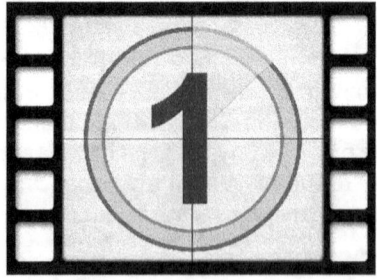

Photo by Antonio Nunes

Cancer:Back Off the Ropes- Thursday, June 18, 2009

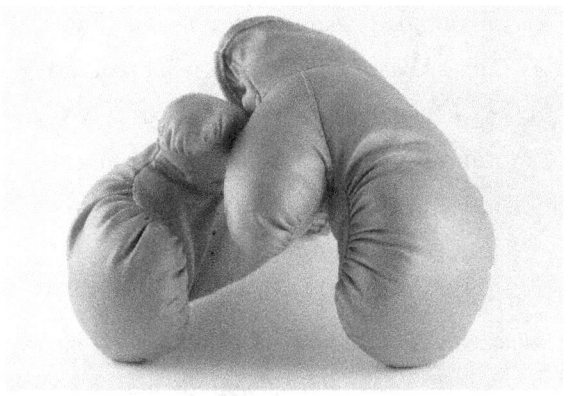

Photo by Adrian Hughes

That damn dragon sucker punched me, but the count was only 8, I'm up on my knees and starting to stand again. I remembered a song today that 'Mas and I sang together that was perfect for where I need to be now.

Bring it on!

by Steven Curtis Chapman

I didn't come lookingʹ for trouble

And I don't want to fight needlessly

But I'm not gonna hide in a bubble

If trouble comes for me

I can feel my heart beating faster

I can tell something's coming down

But if it's gonna make me grow stronger then Bring it on

Let the lightning flash, let the thunder roll,

let the storm winds blow

Bring it on

Let the trouble come, let the hard rain fall,

Afternoons with Ivy

let it make me strong

Bring it on

Now, maybe you're thinkin' I'm crazy

And maybe I need to explain some things

'Cause I know I've got an enemy waiting

Who wants to bring me pain

But what he never seems to remember

What he means for evil God works for good

So I will not retreat or surrender

Bring it on

Let the lightning flash, let the thunder roll,

let the storm winds blow Bring it on

Let the trouble come, let the hard rain fall,

let it make me strong, Bring it on.

Now, I don't want to sound like some hero

'Cause it's God alone that my hope is in

But I'm not gonna run from the very things

That would drive me closer to Him

So bring it on

Let the lightning flash, let the thunder roll,

let the storm winds blow

Bring it on

Let the trouble come, let it make me fall

on the One who's strong

Bring it on

Let the lightning flash, let the thunder roll,

let the storm winds blow

Bring it on

Let me be made weak so I'll know the strength

of the One who's strong

Bring it on

Cancer: Back Off the Ropes

The times they are a-changin'. Sunday I turned a corner. Since Sunday I have been slowly getting back on my feet. That dragon is about to get a southpaw cross. Even if I lose this battle, I'm going out swinging because that's my style. Hello there Dragon, Let's dance!

As I extended my arm for the blood draws today I let it be known that I wanted a copy of the results mailed to me. Before I took my seat on that ice cold metal table for the MUGA scan, I made sure she would make TWO copies, one of which was for me. She offered to have it for me tomorrow. "I want the written report too". When she said I would have to get that from my doctor, I asked when he would have it. A couple days? No problem. I'll be back in two days to get both of them. See ya then! Tuesday the prognostic markers gave me my first ray of sunshine thus far. Finally, some good news. The PR and ER markers were positive. That means that the estrogen in my body is fueling the cancer. There are drugs that can block the cancer's access to that fuel, and we can starve this dragon to death.

I called a friend today, another professional woman, who has recently been here facing her own dragon. She's a one year survivor. I listened as she described how she took her dragon head on, calling the shots as she steamrollered into the lair. I felt a sardonic smile start to twitch at the corner of my mouth. YES! That's the attitude I'm missing. Like osmosis, I could feel her confidence and determination transmit through the phone wires into my ear. Can she bottle that stuff?? I'll take a case of it! By the time we hung up I felt even more empowered. I did some research, called my insurance company and then dialed the surgeon's phone number." I would like you to arrange a second opinion for me in Iowa City," (in our PPO) and I want *this* particular oncologist (Also in our PPO with a 4 star patient rating at a 4 star hospital), please. As always, the surgeon's staff is accommodating and helpful. Confirming that I have about three weeks before chemo therapy should begin, I'm thinking I have just enough time. I know that because of my heart complications, I need the best shot I can get, and I'll only get one. We will certainly meet with the current oncologist again on Tuesday as planned and hear his game plan. I have devised a list of 12 questions for him so far. But I'm not trusting my life to any one individual. In God we trust, all others...

These times, they *have* to change if I'm going to flatten that Dragon on her kiester. She may get me on the ropes again, but she has to get a 10-count before she wins.

Today I ate some green stuff out of a garden with my supper, a gift from a friend. I added some "healthy" salad dressing from that same friend. Tomorrow another friend is bringing me a lunch of assorted edible goodies that I am not going to ask questions about until *after* I have tasted it. Now

I'm getting ready to take my nighttime walk with 'Mas. All fighters train before they get into the ring. I am in training... Because the times. they are a-changing and I'm gearing for a fight.

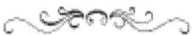

The goal is to live a full, productive life even with all that ambiguity. No matter what happens, whether the cancer never flares up again or whether you die, the important thing is that the days that you have had you will have lived.

~ Gilda Radner

Nickelback : If Today Was Your Last Day Lyrics

My best friend gave me the best advice
He said each day's a gift and not a given right
Leave no stone unturned, leave your fears behind And try to take the path less
traveled by. That first step you take is the longest stride
CHORUS
If today was your last day
And tomorrow was too late
Could you say goodbye to yesterday?
Would you live each moment like your last?
Leave old pictures in the past
Donate every dime you have?
If today was your last day
Against the grain should be a way of life
What's worth the prize is always worth the fight. Every second counts 'cause there's no
second try. So live like you'll never live it twice
Don't take the free ride in your own life
Would you call old friends you never see? Reminisce old memories
Would you forgive your enemies?
Would you find that one you're dreamin' of, swear up and down to God above
That you finally fall in love
If today was your last day
If today was your last day
Would you make your mark by mending a broken heart? You know it's never too late
to shoot for the stars, Regardless of who you are, So do whatever it takes
'Cause you can't rewind a moment in this life. Let nothin' stand in your way
Cause the hands of time are never on your side

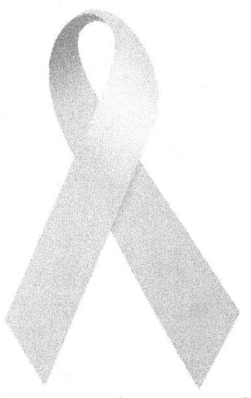

Photo by Amy Dunn

Yesterday I bought a magnetic pink ribbon that says "survivor" and secured it to my front quarter panel of my car. For some reason, it wasn't just an ordinary purchase. I perused the selections carefully. There were actually three options. One said nothing, one promoted early detection, and one said "survivor". My eyes gravitated toward the "survivor" ribbon, but like a child whose hand just got caught in the cookie jar, I wasn't sure if I should. I walked away from the booth, but eventually came back to it. I found my husband, the banker for the day, and hit him up for $4. Then I asked him to accompany me to that first booth where we discussed which ribbon to get.

"Do you think the survivor ribbon is too presumptuous on my part?" I asked. 'Mas suggested that if I were uncomfortable with that choice I could choose one of the other ones. Then he reminded me of what another survivor had recently said to me..."You are a survivor the moment the doctor told you that you had cancer." I remembered that too. It occurred to me that if I didn't beat this, it became a simple matter of pulling that ribbon off of my car. Today it occurs to me that if I don't make it, the ribbon can be placed on 'Mas' car, because he then must survive the outcome, and like me, I expect him to fight his despair with a vengeance.

People who beat cancer are not the only survivors. Win or lose, their families are just as locked in battle, and just as victimized by it. If someone dies, the family is left to reassemble the jigsaw fragments of their lives in order to survive the outcome. The ribbon can serve as a legacy to the battle that ensued, and the exhaustive effort I gave to defeat my dragon.

My thoughts have wandered to other places as well. As various survivors and their families contact me with encouraging words, I begin to realize a few less pleasant character traits about myself. Where was I when they were going through their battle? Was I there in a supportive way? Did I know it at all? Did I do more than give patronizing acknowledgment to their trials? Did I do enough? Funny how walking in someone else's moccasins changes your perspective in such a humbling way. My heart is heavy for the ones I may have inadvertently slighted when they needed me most. If I had only called more often.

If only I had sent more cards. If only I had visited them more. Hindsight is often 20/20, and there is nothing I can do about that. I can only be grateful that they have used their experiences to help the people who follow, like me. I have vowed to myself that if I slay this dragon, I will remember this experience and use it to be more compassionate, more thoughtful, and more supportive in the future.

There are certain life lessons that I am already learning in this process. Some of them are the subtle sorts of things that I was just too busy to absorb before it started. One of those lessons is, in fact, just being too busy. I know that God plans to forcibly slow me down once the chemo starts. Another is choosing priorities. I've also learned that I have friends who really do care, and are willing to demonstrate it by going the extra mile for me. Some of these lessons would not be accomplished had it not been for this dragon nipping at my heels. God can even use dragons to glorify himself.

On Monday I will go and retrieve the test results of last Thursday. On Tuesday, we will meet again with the oncologist. My incision is healing well, and I can almost straighten my arm over my head. I anticipate that the chemotherapy I am dreading is about two weeks out. Time flies when you are NOT having fun.

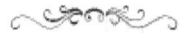

Women agonize... over cancer; we take as a personal threat the lump in every friend's breast.
~ Martha Weinman Lear, *Heartsounds*

Cancer:The Bumpy Ride Ahead-
Tuesday, June 23, 2009

(*Author's Note: what follows represents my first impressions of the oncologist at a time when my head was reeling with changes too fast for me to keep pace with! My oncologist turned out to be a compassionate man and time improved our communication*) In the movie, *All About Eve*, Betty Davis said, "Fasten your seat belts, it's going to be a bumpy night." If I change the word "night" to be "ride", I think the quote is appropriate here. Once the lumpectomy and pathology report became past tense, the week that followed seemed comparatively slow while we waited on those prognostic markers and for my body to adequately heal.

Like an episode of Star Trek, today we just moved back into warp speed and both 'Mas and I feel a bit overwhelmed! With the MUGA scan behind us, we revisited the oncologist, expecting to move forward in this journey we have embarked upon, and we were not disappointed.

We were ushered into the inner office quickly. I mentally checked my oncologist grade book next to promptness and took my seat in the "chair on the left", while I checked the time on my cell phone and wondered if he would pass the secondary promptness test as well. So often I have been directed into a doctor's "inner sanctum" to wait even longer, without benefit of magazines or television to pass the time. What's up with that? I'm thinking that 30 minutes should be sufficient for *both* in order to get an "A" on that page of the exam. After a short time I heard him outside the door, and decided he would get an overall "B" for his effort.

I determined that the polite approach was to hear what he had to say first, before hammering him with my list of 20 questions. The HER2 report was faxed to him almost immediately, so that became our starting point. According to the Miami Molecular lab, my HER2 was actually negative. For anyone but me that might of been a bad thing, but as usual, leave it to me to be the rebel! A positive HER2 would have called for a specific drug that would be very hard on my already compromised heart, greatly limiting my options.

That brought us to the MUGA scan results which came as no great surprise to me. Pardon me if I am too technical here but I do have folks with a medical background reading this blog, so for their benefit, my ejection fraction was 81%. To you and me that means my heart doesn't rest well, and it is enlarged and stiffened. (sort of matches my neck!) A phrase that most will recognize: cardiomyopathy. I'll let you Google that one for yourself! I have been

Googling my fingers to the bone! To be even more precise, I have diastolic congestive heart failure. (Whoopee! Big word that simply means my heart is crappy) That brings us to treatment choices, and the oncologist indicated that if I want him to bypass caution with regard to the risk to my heart, he would proceed with the strongest chemo that would give my survival the greatest opportunity....uh, no. It doesn't make a lot of sense to me to endure the trauma of chemo only to cause a potential sudden cardiac death because of it. In my play book, the objective of the game is to LIVE. Swapping the risk of one form of death for another doesn't sound like a good game plan to me. So I chose the less risky form of chemo cocktail. Fill 'er up, Joe!

Ahh but the story doesn't end there. (you really didn't think it would, did you?) The less risky version of the chemo treatment, while kinder to my heart, is also kinder to the cancer cells. What could have been an 80% survival rate of cancer death on the stronger, harsher drug now drops to less than 60%. But at least that beats my odds if I skip the chemo, which would drop the statistics to 30%. I will have four to six treatments, each lasting up to four hours, once every three weeks for the next 5 months IF I handle it well enough, at which time the radiation phase will begin.

He took a gander at my yellow legal pad and said, "I didn't allocate enough time to answer your questions." It must have been a Kodak moment as my eyebrows shot up, and according to 'Mas, I presented my best "Evil Eye Fleegle". Those of you who are my age might remember back to 1952, when a character named Evil Eye Fleegle appeared on the Fearless Fosdick TV show. (no smart remarks from the peanut gallery!) If you are so old that your memory needs a little jog:

"EVIL-EYE FLEEGLE had a unique and terrifying skill. When he concentrated, destructive rays emitted from his eyeballs. An ordinary "whammy" could knock a grown man senseless. A "double whammy" could fell a skyscraper, leaving Evil-Eye exhausted. His dreaded "quadruple whammy" could melt a battleship but almost kill Fleegle himself.

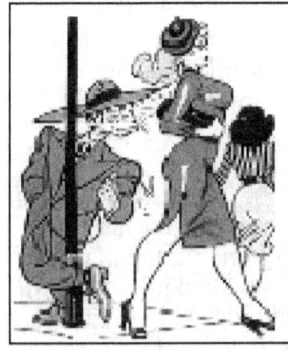

I'm thinking that my glance rated at least a double whammy. As the steel door of communication slammed shut from my side, the key clinked loudly in the lock, the doctor must have noticed how the room temperature dropped to sub-zero in spite of the heat, because he offered to answer a *couple* of general questions before he sent in his nurse to answer any others. "Never mind," responded the Ice Queen. "I didn't realize that the nurse had taken the same college courses that you did." Is that frost on that window? Although I couldn't see his breath as he responded, he did hustle to let me know that he didn't want to rush me, so I could go ahead and ask my questions. I gave him a half of a point for realizing that he had dug himself a deep hole, and another 1/2 point for being smart enough to back peddle out of it. Nevertheless, I did not intend to make his absolution easy. "Never mind," I hissed. "I'll ask the nurse my questions, and we'll see how many she can answer. Then if she can't, I'll make an appointment and come back just to ask them of you."

"Oh, by the way," (left jab coming) "Here is an article about the negative effects of splenda on chemotherapy patients. Since I am a diabetic, and I want to get my diabetes under control in preparation for an eventual pet scan, should I go easy on the splenda? I doubt if your nurse is up on this one." After explaining to him that splenda was that little yellow packet that people poured into their coffee, he confessed that he was unaware of this research. "That's okay, this is your copy, and you may have it to read if you would like." (Don't they have splenda in Greece?)

I made sure he understood that this is MY life and death we are talking about, I WILL be a part of this process, and I need to be able to understand what he is doing to me if I am going to trust him at all. I asked about two drugs that I had researched. He was surprised that I knew to ask about them at all. I'm thinking that if he knew me, he would know this is precisely what I would do. After he left the office, I thought to myself that we are both lucky he didn't flunk the test today. If he had not softened his approach, our professional relationship would have ended. He would have lost a client, and I would have had to delay treatment even longer while I found a new oncologist.

The next topic was picc or port? Paper or plastic? Since repeated IV's are hard on the veins, and bad veins make for painful IV's, the issue becomes that of inserting a way that the IV's can be injected more easily. A couple of survivor friends of mine had already warned me to choose port. A bit more invasive procedure, it offered better long term results. My primary question was this, "can I still use my hot tub with a picc?" The answer was no, so my decision became simple. I already have to leave the right arm out of the water, so winter tubbing is now officially a thing of the past. (that arm will freeze at 20 degrees without benefit of 102 degree water!) With a picc line, I would be unable to put the left arm into the water as well! Hot tubbing is a big part of our "quiet together" time, and a tradition that has been upheld for several years between 'Mas and I. That's one small constant that I would like to keep.

After a short discussion with the nurse about the sordid details of chemotherapy side effects and some homework reading for me, we proceeded to the front desk while the receptionist scrutinized the calendar. The date of June 30 was penciled in for the first chemotherapy, providing we could get the port in quickly enough. That added a little unexpected side trip to our homeward commute for a visit with the surgeon. July 1 would be a trip back for a shot that I could not expediently obtain the same day as the chemo. That is how the treatment will progress...Tuesday is the chemo, Wednesday is the trip back for the shot. Notice how there is no Thursday in this equation? In the car, on the way to the surgeon's office, 'Mas and I agreed that we were a bit overwhelmed. The sudden speed of events was daunting and seemed surreal. I felt myself tense at the prospect of those side effects and sure enough, at my feet, my dragon lay curled with one yellow eye cracked while a sneer curled her lips. I delivered a swift kick to her nose and she responded with a raspy ribbon of flame that singed my shoe. Damned annoying dragon!

Onward to Betty's wig shop to pick up a wig. 'Mas still likes it, so I guess it will do. The lady gave me a receipt for my "cranial prosthesis", and reminded me to submit it to the insurance. I'm pretty sure they aren't paying for that one! As instructed, I called the insurance company last week to ask if they covered a "cranial prosthesis". I had to explain what that was, and the answer was no. I doubt if attaching an Rx to it is going to make any difference.

Comfort Food! Since nobody else was looking, 'Mas and I pulled the car into IHOP for a tasty lunch of carbs. I think I was okay with the scrambled eggs and fried ham, but maybe the hash browns were a bit much, and no doubt the cream cheese stuffed french toast was over the top. But hey! Like any good carb junkie, I compensated my indulgence with a diet coke! Name me an overweight woman who doesn't acknowledge a food binge with a diet drink! I considered the dragon nestled on the floor of my car, but then decided "ta heck with her! She can starve!"

Soon, the car is going to have the route to Hammond Henry memorized. We won't even need to steer the wheel! We had several stops to make here. One to the GP about adjusting my diabetic medicine, one to the surgeon to schedule putting in the port, and one to the radiology department to pick up my CD of the MUGA scan. As usual, the surgeon's nurse Ione bent over backwards to accommodate our unexpected request. Her first offering was on Thursday. Thursday?? Not Thursday! We aren't doing any more Thursdays! With a short negotiation, the procedure was slated for next Monday morning. She assured me that I would get a good dose of lala drugs to satisfy my fears of masochistic tendencies. I made a mental note to tell anyone that asked me about Dr. Atwell that I would give him a high recommendation.

Headed back to Kewanee, we took a short detour to Darla, our hairdresser. I showed her the wig and we made a plan to deal with the loss of my hair. My intent was to cut it short when I started chemo, but the time constrains aren't going to allow that. Plan B: when my hair begins to fall out, (probably in about 3 weeks) she will shave it off for me. We discussed eyebrows and eyelashes, and how we would deal with those things as well. Earlier today I did some research about eyebrows. I nearly fell off my chair when I learned that there is such a thing as "eyebrow wigs". I kid you not! As I laughed out loud to myself, I wondered if people would notice a bad eyebrow wig the way they notice a bad toupee. Still makes me laugh at the prospect. I decided I would settle for something simpler and a bit more old fashioned.

I wonder how folks would react if I show up at church with some Groucho Marx glasses? You know, the ones with the big bushy eyebrows and nose attached! At least I would have eyebrows! What could be funny is the look on their faces as they struggle to be PC with the cancer victim while trying to maintain a straight face. Maybe I should have 'Mas hide around a corner, so he could capture those moments on the camera!

With a double mastectomy potentially in the offing, I asked 'Mas what size he would like. LOL! Someone told me the other day that in the case of only one breast reconstruction it is required to "tweak" the real remaining breast because it sags with age, while the artificial breast remains "perky". Something about that visual cracks me up. Sorry, I warned you that my sense of humor would become even more twisted

Once we reached Manchester Drive, we drove passed our house and directly to my best friend Linda's house, a few doors up the street. We filled her in on the game plan, discussed how best to utilize the offers for rides and foods, reaffirmed her position as "point" person, and sealed the deal with some soda. Home once again, I wandered into my usual place in the office, and began to update this blog.

I must admit that I am afraid of chemo. I'm also afraid of the array of needles that are about to become a normal part of my future. I have never enjoyed hugging the porcelain pedestal while calling the Irish, (O'Rourke) even when I put myself there by my own volition with a zesty bottle of raspberry ripple! but after those eyebrow wigs, I know that I still have my sense of humor, and each day my determination grows. That dragon is still hanging out, but she's been bored this past week, and has had plenty of time to contemplate what she will do when she loses her job here.

I think that it can safely be said that I am getting my TUDE (attitude) back, and while it may not be my most endearing quality, I think that it will serve me well in this situation. I welcome those moments when my laughter replaces my tears. I've never liked crying much, especially around a dragon! And Rambo-mode works well for subduing fear. They are the tools of the trade when it comes to my life. I hope that the side effects of the chemo don't throw me under the bus.

Seems to me that our greatest fear is the unknown, and that most often, we tend to choose unacceptably familiar to the question mark that best represents the alternative. But if I'm going to fight this dragon, I'm going to fight to win, and I will pour all of me into the effort. If I go out, it will be swinging! And as the "stepping into the ring" video (Nicole Johnson) so aptly pointed out, cancer cannot follow me to the grave. She can kill my body, but she can't kill my spirit. Ding! Ding!

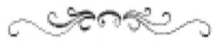

> # Do not be afraid of tomorrow; for God is already there.
>
> ## ~Author Unknown

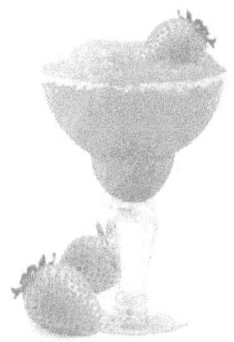

I heard a new phrase today, and I've decided to keep it. The infusion center is notoriously known as the "Cocktail lounge" by those who frequent it. I've always enjoyed a good play on words, so I will adopt this catchy phrase, wishing I had been the clever person who thought of it. There is just so much humor that can be adapted to it! Maybe the phrase can serve to override some of the fear that I am attaching to chemotherapy.

"Bartender, I would like a TC cocktail please, and make it neat!". Doesn't that sound less intimidating than the terms infusion center and chemotherapy? Truth be known, I don't think there will be anything neat about it. "Give me a shot with that!". "I would like to try a nice port". I'm guaranteed to get the shot, and the port will hopefully spare my veins a considerable amount of discomfort.

I think that part of the dread surrounding chemotherapy is that you have no way to anticipate what will happen because it affects everyone differently. You can't actually brace yourself for it. I find myself frantically working to eliminate a list of projects from my desk because I'm not sure if I will become too sick to finish them, and we have contractual obligations to our clients. I can't *plan* anything because I don't know if I will be too busy holding my head over a bucket. Life is moving at warp speed right now, and yet, aside from work load, my world seems to have skidded to a screeching halt. I'm afraid to commit to much of anything for fear that I won't be able to follow it through. I have become a responsible person in my aging years, and if I say I am going to do something, I do it. Suddenly, contrary to my own will, I don't know if I can. Plans that have been in the works for months are now suspended, perilously waiting for the air current to move them one direction or the other. I'm never going to be nominated for any awards of my organizational skills, but at least I had a plan! Now I don't even seem to have that beyond getting through today to see tomorrow.

you couldn't motivate me any other way, add a generous helping of guilt. I am programmed to pick up guilt. Guilt trips have taken me around the world and back. I've spent years undoing the guilt program. My dragon loves guilt. Now here I am, packing my bags for a series of new guilt trips. Being unable to fulfill my jobs around the house will give me guilt. Being unable to keep up my usual standards for our business will award heaps of guilt. Seeing my husband try to do both my work and his own...guilt. Imposing on friends to give me rides to chemo...guilt. The inability to entertain people whose company I normally enjoy...guilt. Saying no when I really want to say yes...more guilt. Most of all, asking friends to do simple tasks that I just cannot seem to get done will make me feel horribly guilty. It occurs to me that there are as many emotional side effects to cancer as there are physical ones!

Yes, I know that friends are offering, and that they want to help. I appreciate them more than they could ever know. But I still feel guilty. Guilty because I may not be able to do the things that I have always done for myself. Maybe I'll be one of the lucky ones who sails through chemo with nary a hitch. That would be nice, of course, but I do not believe it for a moment and I sure as heck won't count on it.

Funny how life teaches us new meanings for old terms. A couple of weeks ago I realized that I'm a "fixer". When I encounter a problem, my instincts are to fix it, but it doesn't always work. I can't fix this. I just realized that I am also a "bracer". I don't live in the moment. I brace for what is coming next, whether I need to or not. I can't brace for chemotherapy. It's this invisible, elusive adversary that waits for me around the next corner. Ah, my dragon will love chemotherapy. My dragon loves to lurk in dark places that stink of fear. In my ongoing bout with my dragon, I won round one. Now I'm resting nervously on a stool in the corner, watching the referee raising the hammer to the bell for round 2. My dragon paces with anticipation, sizing me up, strategically hunting for the best place to land her next blow. Her tail is fidgeting restlessly. Geez! Doesn't she ever get tired?? I think part of her strategy is to keep hitting me so fast that I don't have time to think or regroup. Maybe she figures that if she keeps me in a dead run, she can wear me down easier and maybe she'll be right. But not today. Today I will spar with her even though I won't taunt back. Today I will duck and weave and keep moving around that canvas ring, so that she isn't able to get me on the ropes. Guilt and fear give her an advantage, but it doesn't guarantee her a victory.

Cancer: Cocktail Anyone?

Here's an idea! Hey dragon! Want to join me for a cocktail? I won't tell her that the cocktail she is served is supposed to be lethal for her. I think that I will enjoy seeing her writhe in pain. Suddenly I envision an old movie or play wherein the bad guy slips the good guy a poisonous drink, only to smile sardonically as the poor schmuck realizes his fate, grabs his throat, and crumples to the floor in a dead heap. Only in my vision, the good guy (me) serves up the sauce. My smile is likely to be just as twisted.

Hmm, I kind of like that story...Bartender, make it a double!

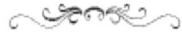

My veins are filled, once a week with a Neapolitan carpet cleaner stilled from the Adriatic and I am as bald as an egg. However I still get around and am mean to cats.

~John Cheever

Cancer: She Waits- Saturday, June 27, 2009

There is an old cliché', "you can never go home again". In many ways, cancer makes this so. My life will never be the same again. There is no turning back and there is nothing that I can do about it.

In two days we round another corner. Each corner is scarier than the last. Each corner is harder to face. With each turn the stakes become higher. Like water smoothes granite, cancer wears me down.

I think that I must have inkling, just an inkling, of how the man of Christ must have felt in the Garden of Gethsemane about what lay ahead of Him. He must have been afraid, like I am afraid. He must have known dread like I am feeling dread. He must have felt powerless like I am feeling powerless. Certainly, He must have felt alone, like I feel alone, because no one could go in His place. This isn't the movies, and there is no stand-in waiting in the wings to take my place when the scene becomes too dangerous to risk its star.

As the minutes tick by, and daylight wanes to dusk my dragon takes her position directly behind me, stalking me, and patiently waiting for my resolve to dissolve into a puddle of sweat at my feet. She says nothing. There are no flames tickling my neck, no smoke clouding my view. She just watches and waits quietly. She knows that I am terrified. She can smell my fear. There is no need to taunt me and she knows it. She is confident while I am not.

I can feel her steely gaze boring into my back. I could see her shadow loom beside me in the glare of the streetlight as we took our nightly walk. She is there and she is waiting. I know that her yellow eyes are staring at me because I have seen them before. I am prey and she is the predator.

Like Jesus did so many centuries before me, I want to beg God to take this away. Give me my life back! Don't make me go through this. Please, reconsider! But for whatever reason, this is my lot. This is the hand that I have been dealt, and I must see it through. I don't understand why this is happening to me. I guess I don't have to understand. It just is. It is times such as these when I can only trust that God is in control and He knows what He is doing. Sometimes that is a comfort, but not this night. This night I am afraid and she is waiting. This night I am no longer a strong woman. This night I am a little girl, seeking a skirt tail to hide behind. This night I desperately yearn to hear my daddy's voice tell me that everything will all be alright. It's been so long since I have heard his voice. Would I remember it? This night I am afraid of the darkness at the top of the stairs. This night a large, green, scaly Bogeyman is stalking me. This is a night for sleeping with the light on.

I want to be brave. I try to be the warrior. But sometimes I feel so small, and this is one of those times. Two steps forward, one step back. I strive to move forward, but like a soldier trudging through mud up to his knees, my pack is weighing me down, and that backpack is full of fear, apprehension, dread, and anxiety. Like quicksand it threatens to suck me under. All the while, my dragon waits quietly and watches me struggle like a drowning man.

Will I still be me after they pump that poison into my veins? Will it hurt? Will my hair fall out in large clumps? Or will it be more subtle? How will I feel when I gaze in the mirror? Will I recognize me? Will I be sick everyday? Or just some days? Will my bones ache as the drugs chase the cancer through them? If my life is going to change, who will I become? Will I remember who I was?

No, I can never go home again. At least not home as I knew it before this cancer. The house will be the same, the street will look the same, the people will act the same, but I will be forever changed. No one survives a war unscathed. There are always casualties. I will never view life in quite the same way I used to. Some of those changes will be good changes. Some will not. I can only hope that the new me will be an improved version of the old me when the smoke finally clears.

But until then I must get through *this* night. This night I am afraid and she is watching.

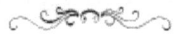

Cancer: A Port in Any Storm-

It's so great that God knows what I need before I do! This weekend held a lot of stress for us about the upcoming procedures and chemotherapy and my dragon was never very far away. I had contacted my son and his family requesting an audience while I was still well enough to enjoy the visit. I had no idea what a blessed distraction they would be. I always enjoy spending time with them, and this visit was a special treat.

The house was alive with warmth. There was laughter and lots of hugs. It was nice to awaken to the sounds of yawning and fresh perked coffee. As usual, our time together flew by and before I realized it, the weekend had mostly passed by with nary a dark cloud. When I made my request, it hadn't crossed my mind that their presence would become such an effective tool at keeping my dragon at bay. God knew, and he wasn't done yet.

Their car had barely left our driveway when another one replaced it. Some weeks back, before chemo arrangements had been made, we invited some good friends from Texas visiting their local family to use our guestroom. Lisa and Mike had been church friends before they ever moved to Texas, and Lisa had just had a breast cancer scare of her own in January. Lucky for her, it was only a scare, but the experience put us on a familiar page, and she has become my long distance chemo buddy. Before nightfall, they arrived and my dragon was denied yet another opportunity to badger me. We talked well into the night and by morning, we were up and on our way to the hospital to have the port inserted.

I was scheduled for surgery at 11, but they wanted me there a little early to check my sugar levels. As usual, they were too high. I must say that Genesis East could use a makeover on how things operate over there. Delays are somewhat unavoidable and I understood that. My surgery got delayed until about 4pm! But more disconcerting were the oversights. Things like needing to remind the staff to give me the insulin on several occasions, and reminding at least 5 different nurses about my allergy to tape only to find that they dressed the wound with standard tape anyway. (I was unconscious, so couldn't remind them that time). The wound had to be completely redone with the paper tape.

My surgery actually went without a hitch, but by the time I got out of surgery, we hadn't eaten in 15 hours, so we were both ravenous! I was served 4 graham crackers, 4 soda crackers along with a glass of sierra mist. Poor 'Mas passed on those since he figured I would need the sustenance. That was an appetizer! I'm talking HUNGRY! Hospital checkouts always seem to take longer than they should, and my growling stomach began to become a growling woman in a hurry to find a restaurant on the route home!

The closest restaurant on the route home turned out to be a KFC. Okay, not the best diet, but I figured I had earned a hot meal and by this point I wasn't very picky! We finally arrived home at around 10pm.

Once home, it occurred to me that God was ahead of me again. While a 5 hour delay might have been an annoying inconvenience, the end result that it was late and I was tired. My thoughts, once again, were distracted from my fears, and my snugly bed took second place on my priority list. The day had been exhausting, and sleep came quickly. As we reviewed our day, we noticed how God had kept us distracted throughout the course of the 3 days preceding the chemotherapy. My dragon had not even made it through the front door. Thank you God, for being so smart and seeing to the need that I didn't even know I had.

I have a new appreciation for the word "distraction". I also have a new list of ways to conjure it up. More new lessons for a cancer process that offers few rewards. I now know that I can invoke distraction through watching a movie, and sharing fellowship with much loved family and friends. I have always enjoyed those things, but failed to realize the deeper significance that they offer. And I will remember this lesson for the future, when someone that I love is dealing with a crisis. I will make it my goal to just "be there", to spend some time with them and help distract them from the painful thoughts and fears that haunt them. I will help keep their dragons away. I now have tools that I didn't know I had when I find myself in those awkward moments when comforting words escape me. I have learned that there is a "port" for every storm.

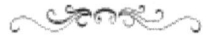

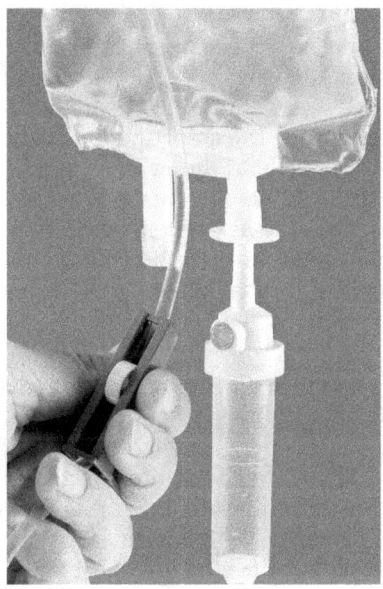

Photo by Anna Schram

Today was a huge day for us. We were now facing some very large fears. All the horror stories we had heard about chemotherapy were about to be put to the test.

I woke to a sore port, which I had been told to expect. It wasn't hurting so much I couldn't handle it, but I knew that they were going to be messing with it, so I allowed myself to take a vicodin to keep irritation to a minimum. I was also nervous, so I popped a couple of my lorazepam to settle my jangled nerves. That put me in pretty good shape for the trip to the cocktail lounge.

My appointment was at 10:15 and I was the first patient to be ushered into the cocktail lounge. There were four comfortable recliners at the ready, and I had my choice of seats. We picked one with a nice view of the plasma television and I arranged my chemo bag next to my chair. My research had revealed some handy tips which I had acted upon, so I came prepared with a bag containing some essentials. Before we left the house, my chemo buddy had brought me a warm blanket and matching pillow. I remembered how cold the air-conditioning was when we were there the last time, so I gratefully loaded the ensemble into the car. Cathy reminded me to carry a container in the event that I got sick during the car ride, a reminder that I appreciated. I hadn't thought of that one, and I didn't savor the idea of getting sick in the new Rav. Actually I wasn't as worried about messing up the new car as I dreaded having to clean it up! Thus I was pretty organized for this junket.

I situated myself in my chair of choice, while 'Mas tried to make himself comfortable in the "visitor's" chair. (not nearly as accommodating as mine!) I pulled out my water bottle and pillow. The chemo nurse carried in a variety of clear plastic pouches containing the assortment of antidotes specific to the occasion. There was a steroid (that I didn't want to take at all!), an anti-nausea drug, and some saline. She flushed the port, and then hooked me up to the various concoctions. I was suddenly grateful for the port. They had left the needle in place from the surgery the night before so that there wouldn't be a need to poke around what was already a sore place. That process went without a hitch.

I noticed that one of the meds made my foot itch, but when the chemo nurse introduced the vial of benadryl, the itching stopped and I got sleepy. Benadryl always makes me sleepy. I dozed off and on. The next vial to be added was the taxotere. The first time taxotere is administered, it can cause an allergic reaction, so we were all watching for it. I could feel the coolness of each drug as it entered the port. My heart did begin to race when the taxotere was administered, but the atenolol that I take for my heart normally prevents the heart rate from increasing over a certain level, so it didn't get very far. My BP remained normal with only a tiny elevation. I did feel some pressure on my heart that was different than usual, so the chemo nurse slowed down the taxotere drip and added some more benadryl. That seemed to address the problem as well as lengthen the process, but I was back to sleep quickly.

The cytoxin was saved for last. But again, I seemed to tolerate it well. During the process, the room quickly filled with other chemo patients, so there was a lot of chitchatting and comparing of notes. The next lady in was having her third chemo cocktail, and she was on the same meds as me. I complimented her on her attractive hair only to learn that it was a wig. She had only lost some of the hair in her eyebrows and lashes, so I felt hopeful about that. She said that she hadn't really had much discomfort at all up to this point, which I felt encouraged to hear. Like me, she had only had the lumpectomy. She was a stage 2 and her cancer had not advanced into her lymph nodes, so she had a better prognosis than me, but I had more interest in her experiences with the chemo.

Cancer: Chemotherapy

We were soon joined by another woman stricken with colon cancer. This was not her first bout with cancer or the chemo, so she was the resident veteran in the group. She wasn't a talker like the first lady and her husband, and spent most of the time buried in a book, but she did eventually open up. The last to enter was another breast cancer patient, who was receiving treatment for her 2nd bout with cancer. Her 2nd bout recurred where the first had been taken out and then spread into her other breast. That made me think about the decision that I am weighing to have a mastectomy in both breasts when we get to that.

The entire process today took 5 hours, but that was a little longer because of the taxotere and shouldn't be quite that lengthy from this point forward. My dragon didn't get to participate today either. Once again, there was plenty of distraction and chatter between dozing that kept her at bay. By the end of my treatment I felt pretty normal, and wondered what all that hubbub had been about.

I was warned that the shot I go back for tomorrow may make me ache, and that the nausea typically doesn't hit for a couple days which is why they gave me the follow-up medication. So I am still not off the hook for ugly side effects, but I am not afraid like I was before today. Leaving the cocktail lounge still being me was helpful. I'm feeling my courage start to return again.

I'm also thinking that those wonderful volunteers who will be driving me to my cocktail lounge may do well to plan a shopping excursion after dropping me off. 'Mas said that the chair he sat in got pretty uncomfortable after all those hours, and the vigil is pretty boring for the visitor. There is a fair amount of cancer talk going on amidst the patients present, and if today was any indication, the men seem to congregate in the other large room.

Pack yourself a snack and bottle of water if you are sticking around, since they don't always have them available. You'll get hungry at lunch time, so you might want to work that into your shopping excursion. I'm apt to sleep on the way home a bit, so if you want to take a friend to shop with, just leave me a place to recline in the car.

Tomorrow, before I get the shot, I have made arrangements for my chemo buddy Lisa to take me to my hairdresser. The next time you see me I will have short hair. Maybe I'll try something really different. If I don't like it, so what? It's going to fall out within a couple weeks anyway, so it's not like the style will be permanent! I'm thinking that my dragon isn't going to have much action tomorrow either. She may have to wait a week or so before she gets another crack at me. At least I HOPE so.

Meanwhile, I will keep listening to my Bring it On video daily. I will keep reminding myself that with God's help, I can do this. And I now have only 5 cocktails to go. Your prayers are working, and God is sticking close to my side. This went WAY easier today than I expected it to, and my apprehension has been replaced by relief. I believe that it is a result of all the prayers and light you are sending my way. Thanks!! And keep it up! If it continues like it is today, I know I can do this, no matter what the outcome might be.

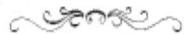

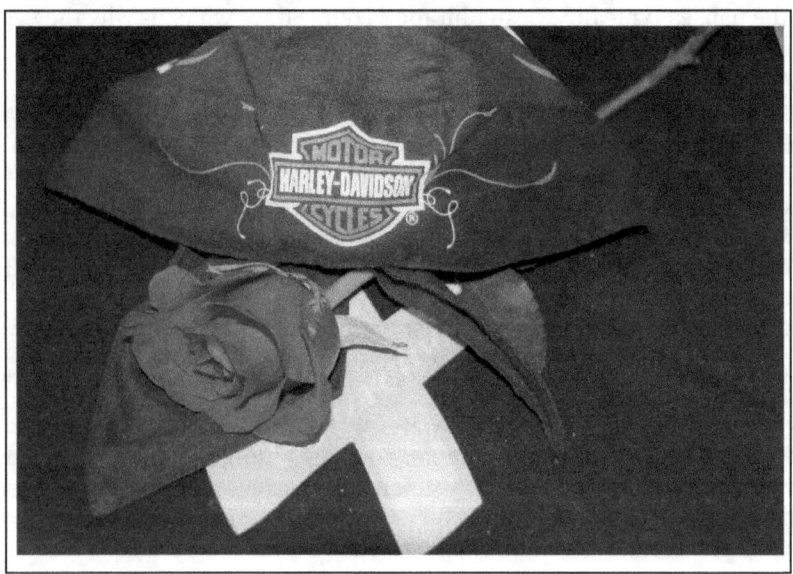

Although difficult to see in this black and white version, when first diagnosed, I looked for a way to define who I was. I needed to feel like I was still me. The Harley Davidson hat represents my toughness; the rose symbolized my femininity, and the survivor ribbon seemed self explanatory to me.

Cancer: Bartender, Gimme Another Shot!-

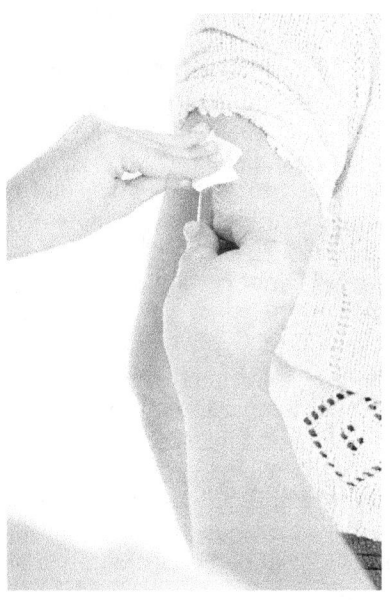

Photo by Daniel Garcia

Each day after chemo I have to return to the scene of the crime for a bone marrow shot. Now returning to a "cocktail lounge" for a "shot" may sound like a fun thing to do on the surface, but it is not. This stinging shot is administered in the fatty part of the arm instead of the port. As it was explained to me, this shot kicks my bone marrow into high gear so that white blood cells can be replenished. Lucky for them I have lots of fatty arm parts to choose from! The text books keep saying that gorillas are our closest ancestors, but aging tells me that, for women at east, Rocky the flying squirrel is a bit more on the mark than any gorilla! Just take a look at Rocky's arms and tell me I'm wrong!

I was feeling pretty good that day, so accompanied by my chemo buddy Lisa, I drove the route myself. We considered hitting the mall only a short distance away, but still a bit fearful of the unfamiliar side effects, I opted against it. It was probably a good thing that I did.

It's hard to say whether my temperament was influenced by the medications, the circumstances or both, but "cranky" would be putting it mildly! I felt tired by the time we got home so I curled up on the couch in the family room. Feeling chilled, I grabbed the fireplace remote in the hopes of diverting some additional heat my way, but it refused to respond as if to say, "Are you crazy?? It's summer!" 'Mas tried to get it lit, but it stubbornly refused. Annoyed, I crawled beneath a blanket and reached for the television remote. At least I could drift off to something on the television. But nooooo, that wasn't happening either. I found myself staring at a blue screen devoid of picture. Once again, poor 'Mas tried to come to the rescue, but the plasma television remained uncooperative. "This is just too much pressure!" I spewed as I tossed aside the blanket and stomped up the steps to our bedroom. Suzy Sunshine was gone on sabbatical and I could have cared less! Hmmm, pity parties...a new wrinkle for me. Complete with black crepe paper, dead flowers and black helium filled balloons sagging to the floor. We *must* be having fun now! I'm not certain if I was more annoyed with the television or myself but I definitely had a TUDE going on.

Crawling beneath the coverlets, I vaguely remember 'Mas announcing that he had finally gotten the television operational again, but I had already begun to succumb to the overwhelming fatigue that was wracking my body. It was still light out but I was already too exhausted to move, much less get up. I noticed that breathing was a bit more difficult, and my port was still sore, but it was the fatigue that seemed to be taking its toll at this juncture. I remember thinking, "Just shoot me now!" before I lapsed into a deep sleep that carried me through to the morning.

The next morning was *Thursday*. That should have been my first clue! I had made a doctor's appointment to get my diabetic meds adjusted. Because I had managed driving so well the previous day, I figured I would be just fine, and didn't want to impose on others to lose their morning carting me over to Geneseo. That was probably my first mistake.

On the trip to Geneseo, I was amazed that I couldn't stop crying. What's up with this?? I couldn't even come up with a logical reason why I was crying, I just kept crying. Depression isn't something that I give in to voluntarily, and I was at a loss with what I should do with this. My nose turned into a faucet, and I kept dabbing my eyes so that I could see through the windshield. I popped a couple of lorazepam and by the time I reached Annawan I could at least see the road clearly, but now my head was loopy and I just didn't feel good at all.

My GP said something about bringing back the spunky me. That obvious, eh? I asked for an anti-depression drug while I was there. I was already adamant about not dealing with these weepies for the next five months! I nixed the idea of zoloft. I had briefly taken that once before, and felt like a zombie. If zoloft is the choice of the oncologist then let him take it. I requested wellbutrin on the advice of a more experienced friend, and I'm hoping that this medication successfully keeps those blues at bay. The surgical nurse made me drink a caffeinated coke before getting behind the wheel. At some point I lost track of my cell phone so I drove by the church to have Gerald call it. I had already retraced my steps so I knew it must be in the car somewhere, but I seemed to be too spacey to figure out where it was. With his help, we found it. By the grace of God I managed to drive back home and crawl back into bed where I spent the remainder of the afternoon.

I didn't realize that through all of this, I was cooking up a temp of 101.3. I remembered that I wasn't supposed to let a temp go unreported, so I phoned the oncologist's office about that. They had me take some ibuprofen and then I was down for the count. The remainder of the day passed by around me. I'm still running a low grade, but it falls within the confines of temperature that I am allowed. I managed to stay awake, (Lord knows how), to watch "Nights in Rodanthe" which was a boring flick. I could have been comatose and still figured out how that movie ended!

Mental note: plan for the worst the day after the shot, and don't make any more appointments on Thursday! Today I'm starting to feel human again, although I notice that my energy level continues to disappoint me. Seems like I work 10 minutes and rest 30. But at least I have been able to get up, so I guess that is a good thing. Even writing this blog seems to require a greater attention span than I have available.

We are going to go to the show uptown and see Ice Age 3 later. I think I feel good enough for that, although the thought of the greasy popcorn that becomes our usual evening fare tends to turn my stomach. Maybe I can sneak in a bag of cherries to munch on. This is the first long holiday we've had in awhile, and we would both very much like to get away. That said, we are considering the new African exhibit that recently opened at the Glen Oak Zoo. There are lots of places to sit, and I would really like to get outside for a day. I'm thinking that the slower pace should work and we would still be close enough to to get home if the need arises.

I'm thinking that I'm apt to disappear between Wednesdays and Thursdays, but not too far away. I'll probably be curled under a blanket somewhere, wasting the most productive part of my day while I saw large logs. Maybe I need to consider a new occupation, like logging. Or maybe Sesame Street could use an extra ZZZZ maker. I'd work cheap!

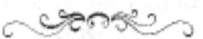

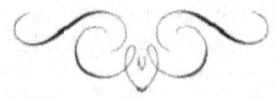

Blessed are You,

Compassionate One,

For giving me

these droplets of

taxotere and cytoxin,

Like refreshing dew

and healing rain,

may they save my life.

Cancer: WipeOut!- Sunday, July 5, 2009

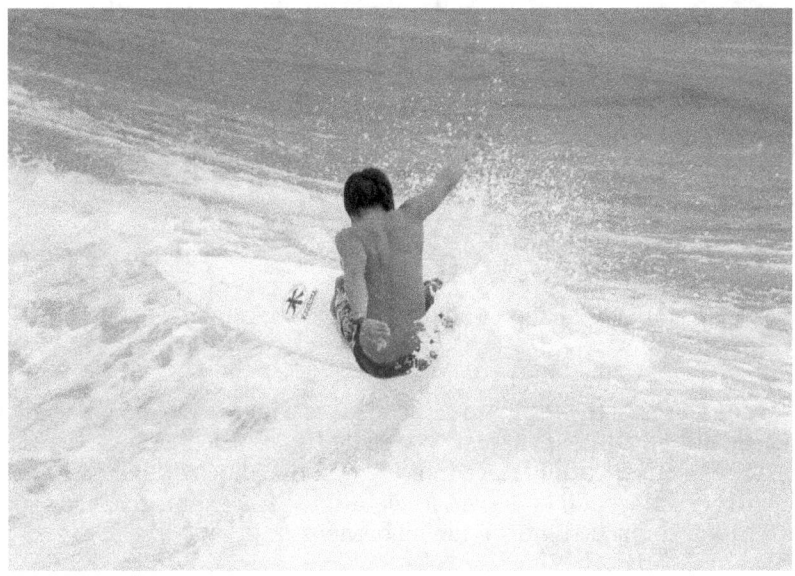

Remember back in the sixties when the Beach Boys were a hot ticket, and surfing was a sport for the "cool" kids? The best Midwesterners could hope for were drive-in movies starring Annette Funicello and Troy Donahue. Well imagine, for a moment, that taunting Beach Boys voice yelling "aaahhhhhhhhh wipe out!" that initiates the song and you will have a pretty good idea of what I looked like by the time we left the zoo today!

Today was a good day, and after yesterday's disappointing rainfall, I was stoked about getting some fresh air and doing something fun for a change. It was the first time since this cancer ordeal started that I was going to act upon my passion for photographing wildlife and I had been looking forward to it! I even managed to make the 8am church service (a rare occasion, indeed) so that we could hit the road to Peoria early. You see, I had planned this little outing carefully. Glen Oak zoo had an exhibit that we hadn't seen yet, was close enough to get home if the occasion warranted it, and far enough away to feel like I was somewhere, anywhere else!

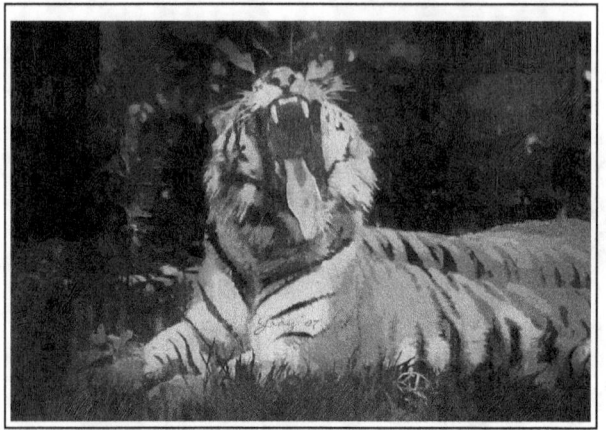

Usually our excursions have me leading the way while 'Mas trudges along behind me. We exchange the usual "Hey, wait up!" or "Hurry up!" banter that aging married folks share as they tag after each other, nursing sore feet and aching joints. Not uncommonly, I eventually lose track of 'Mas, only to retrace my steps and find him perched on a shady park bench, catching his breath. Today was different!

Today it was 'Mas in the lead, retracing his steps, and it was me perched on the bench, not breathless, but just *pooped*! I said, POOPED! As we rounded the bend of the tiger cage I noticed for the first time how few benches were available for resting, and how even fewer seemed to exist in any shady spots. I pretty much stopped at most if not all of them.

In days of old, I would have closed the park, too absorbed with my photography to notice that one of the employees was tapping his toe and frowning at his watch while he waited for me to amble through the exit. Glen Oak is a dual photo opportunity because the botanical garden sits right next door! Typically that would be equivalent to a triple-decker ice cream oozing over the top of a sugar cone! But today it took an enormous amount of stamina just to hobble around this small zoo and there was little energy remaining for walking back to the car (carefully parked right outside the entrance), let alone down the path to the flower gardens!

Dragging my feet slowly, concentrating on one foot in front of the other, I gratefully opened the car door and took my place on the sweltering seat. While 'Mas loaded camera equipment, I took a gander at the time...2:00! Are you kidding me?? We've only been here about 3 hours! 'Mas asked if there was anything else I wanted to do while we were in Peoria, and I was *certain* that there must be, but an honest assessment convinced me that the only thing I really wanted to do was kick off my shoes, curl up on the car seat with my pillow and nap my way back to Kewanee.

There were a couple of other unrelated, but no less annoying things I learned today. Some time back I bought one of those buxton bags like you see on television with the cross-over strap. I'm here to tell you that the bag was junk, but I really liked the cross-over strap and it worked well for carrying my purse with my camera backpack. When I finally ran out of safety pins to hold it together, I tossed that purse into the trash like a basketball player slam-dunking a basketball! It took me *weeks* to find another crossover strapped purse that would hold all the various amenities that I wanted it to hold as well as meet my "skinflint" requirements for cost.

No sooner did I have the new purse, than I found myself unable to use it. My perfect solution became a perfect liability. If I cross it to the right, it rubs my still-sore biopsy wounds uncomfortably. If I cross it to the left, it hurts my port. And this is probably the most money I've EVER spent on a purse because it was such a great solution for me! Is that just wrong or what?? I'm glancing up at God with a stern scowl. You can stop laughing now, it isn't funny!

Last but not least, every time I eat I get stomach cramps. Sometimes I get stomach cramps when I'm *not* eating. So what did they give me for after effects? Anti-nausea pills! I'm not nauseated! I hurt from the stomach cramps! Hey doc, ya got something in that black bag for stomach cramps? Do you have any idea how NOT strategically placed the restrooms are around that zoo? And large stores like super Wal-Mart's should have bathrooms every 30 feet! It's a LONG way from the front of the store to the back of the store! God forbid if I could muster up enough energy to take a hike in the woods! No, no, no...we aren't going to go there!

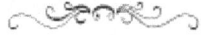

If children have the ability to ignore all odds and percentages, then maybe we can all learn from them. When you think about it, what other choice is there but to hope? We have two options, medically and emotionally: give up, or fight like hell.

~Lance Armstrong

One thing is for certain, cancer is an equalizer. It doesn't matter if you are rich or poor, sophisticated or redneck, educated or stupid, cancer levels the playing field and emotionally speaking, we all end up naked.

This insidious disease exposes the vulnerabilities, weakness of character, and fearfulness of all it infects. It's too overwhelming and goes on too long to maintain a facade. It is what it is, and at some point in time, every cancer victim will feel exposed. I guess that is one of the advantages of having loving friends circle the wagons. Amidst loving friends, there is a certain safety even when naked. There is an understanding that my friends will not exploit my vulnerability and they will hasten to cover my nakedness so that others with less scrupulous intent will not exploit me either. That was not a luxury I had while growing up.

I have always prided myself in being one of the most honest people I know, but even I have a few protective instincts that prevent me from displaying my deepest fears and insecurities. I can't imagine how difficult this nakedness must be for others who are less transparent than I. It troubles me even further that some of those folks lack the support network that I have been blessed with, and as a result, feel even more at risk. Maybe that explains part of the reason I will eventually publish this blog. If I am to be forced into blazing this trail, I hope to sprinkle enough bread crumbs that the next person along the way will find the route a bit easier to traverse.

Common denominators are a part of the nakedness just as veggies are to a salad. Overwhelming fear is a no-brainer. It is experienced by all and overcoming those fears becomes a part of daily life. Anxiety and depression are also a generous portion of the mix. It's what we do with them that makes the difference. My first advice to anyone experiencing this life experience is to circle your wagons. Surround yourself with as many loving family and friends as you can think of.

My second suggestion would be if you lack a faith, get one! Cancer is too great an adversary, and for the most part, steals control. Each cancer patient needs to know that there is something in greater control than the cancer. There needs to be a hope that extends beyond cancer and there needs to be someone or something smart enough to outwit it. That would not be me, and I seriously doubt if it would be you either. There are brilliant minds wrestling with cancer daily that still remain pinned to the mat at the end of the day. They are smarter than me, but still not smart enough. I am of the persuasion that the only one smart enough for that job is God. But if God is not your cup of tea, then find something to sink your hope into.

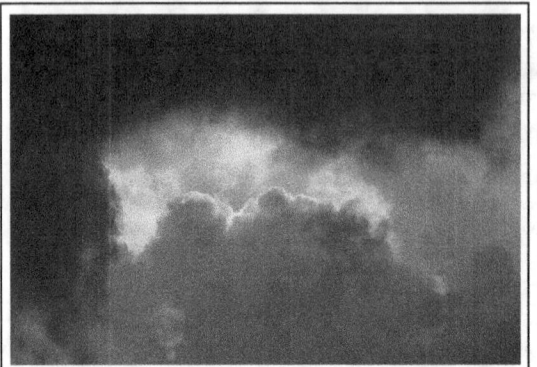

My third piece of sage advice is to scout the horizon for the sliver of silver behind those dark clouds because they are there and they can be priceless. My God always sprinkles them liberally and like a good scout, my binoculars scan the heaven's for them constantly.

A few years ago I lost a young friend named Heidi to this disease. As strange as it might seem, there are days that I can sense Heidi's presence, nudging me and pointing at yet another silver lining. She knows that I am afraid, and she smiles a reassuring smile at me, as if to let me know that everything will work out the way God intends it, and I shouldn't be afraid of that. Heidi dealt with her cancer with the utmost class and dignity. She really raised the bar for me to follow but follow I will. Heidi left behind a legacy of courage and faith as well as a challenge that I must accept. Of course, she already knows what the outcome will be, but she's not telling. It is a well-kept secret between her and God. Her message to me is not about the outcome, but rather the journey. Life may not be a beach, but Heaven certainly is and either way my story ends, I will win. If it is not mine to stay here, then I'll walk along that beach with Heidi, arm in arm, while we laugh and share stories.

I will sprinkle my bread crumbs throughout the course of this blog until such time that we finally reach the outcome, whatever that may be. Hopefully you will find the same humor in this trip that I do, commiserate with my fears, relate to my vulnerabilities, and begin to feel safe in your nakedness. I will also pray that, whoever you are, you will be surrounded by the love of friends and family who will serve to make your journey less perilous.

To those of you who do not face this dragon but know someone who does, don your armor and step between your loved one and the enemy. Whether you choose to pray, send light, provide service, or simply spread encouragement and cheer, join others in that circle. The first attack of the dragon inflicted a near-mortal wound. Your friend is weakened and naked. Your strength and comfort can make all the difference to his or her survival.

So what's become of my dragon, you ask? She's still behind me, but lagging nearly a football field's length at the moment. She's no youngster either, and keeping up with me is proving to be a challenge for her as well. :^) At the moment, her tale's a-draggin! Are you *really* surprised?

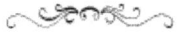

Cancer: Dark Places-Tuesday, July 14, 2009

It's usually in those mindless moments, when my brain briefly stops clamoring about what I haven't done or what I need to do next, that it happens. Since my brain rarely stops the frantic filtering of what is often senseless information, it doesn't happen often, but there are occasional quiet minutes when dark thoughts sneak into dark places.

Typically I am doing something mundane when it happens: a thoughtless process like folding a towel, when my mind begins to wander and I find myself wondering, "who will do this when I'm gone?" The question itself is not a conscious one at first, but like a spaceship re-entering the earth's atmosphere, the sudden jolt back to reality brings the question to the forefront of my mind. Maybe such thoughts are God's way of preventing my denial. Perhaps they serve as a reality check, preparing me for the alternative outcome in the event that the chemotherapy fails to cure me. I'm thinking that just as God prepares us for the physical challenges in our lives, he also directs our thinking so that we are not left unprepared for any situation that arises.

Sometimes I wonder which is more disconcerting...the *act* of dying or the fear of being forgotten. Many a youngster eventually loses the face of a parent or grandparent who passes on. Will they remember my smile? Or how my eyes sparkle when I get excited? Will they think of me when they hear a songbird chirping his melody to the trees? Will they smile when they hear my name? Will they find themselves wishing they could tell me a funny anecdote or something about their day?

I told 'Mas to put a bird feeder with my ashes somewhere, so that I can spend eternity listening to the songbirds I love so much in life. I love waking up each morning to the harmonious twitter outside my window. I fill my feeders often in order to keep the birds near it. Those birds drain those feeders daily, and at times, keeping the feeders full becomes a challenge. The feeders by my ashes will empty quickly too. Will anyone refill them?

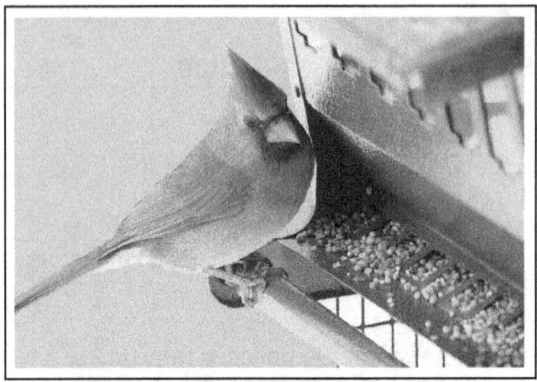

So often I remember time spent with my Grandma, and I spent a lot of time with her, and find myself smiling as I recall something we did together. Many times I wish that I could sit with her again while she shares the vast knowledge that she must have acquired in her lifetime. Sometimes I just miss the comfort of her presence. Ah, but times have changed. Families don't connect the way they used to. Distance prevents that. As a result, grandparents don't get the exposure with grandchildren so bonds don't get cemented like they did between Grandma and me.

In dark places, irrational fears, like mushrooms, are allowed to grow and flourish. The thoughts that we dare not give audience to can prosper. It's probably a good thing that my mind races in infinite circles like a hamster running it's course in its cage because it leaves little opportunity for mindless moments. I wonder why some widowers marry so soon after a life-long relationship? I often wonder why their memories of years spent with someone they loved so much could be so easily replaced. Some say it's not a replacement, but rather a healthy moving on. Maybe, but when they move on with someone else all the remnants of that previous life are erased like words on a blackboard. Pictures are packed away into an attic, and the physical manifestations of a life are removed.

I once had a mother-in-law that remarried each time one of her husbands died. I asked her why she felt compelled to replace each husband with another. Her explanation shed light on a concept that I had never considered. She explained that she experienced happiness in her marriage, so she preferred to live in the state that made her happiest. I had to think on that one awhile. I think I get it, but I don't think it would work for me.

Maybe the reality is that I don't want to move on. Having met my soul mate, I don't believe the experience can be mimicked with anyone else. I don't think I would want it to be and if I believe that, why would I try? Perhaps I would feel differently if I were younger. At this age, I'm ill-prepared to invest the energy that building a relationship takes. I would probably spend too much time comparing to what was. Whatever the reasoning, I prefer to spend my future savoring the experience of my past.

Certainly these are dark thoughts that linger in dark places, but perhaps they are necessary to the *act* of dying. That doesn't make them a bad thing, but rather a necessary thing, because letting go of life is a process and facing the inevitabilities is a part of it. Don't mistake my thoughts as surrender. I'm not done fighting and I'm not giving up. I'm merely acknowledging pieces of a process that I believe we all go through when we are in the act of dying. We all will die sometime, and thus we all will go through this process. The dark places are momentary and fleeting, but they exist and sometimes in the stillness, they just are.

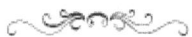

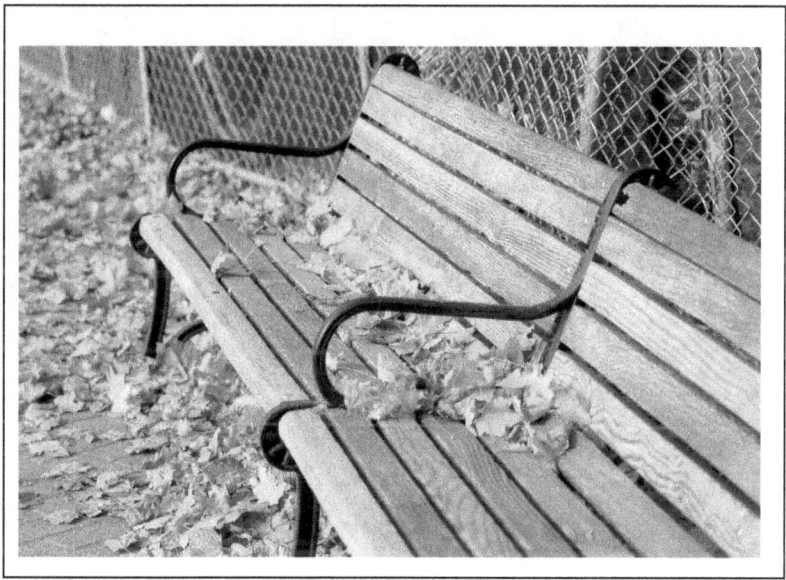

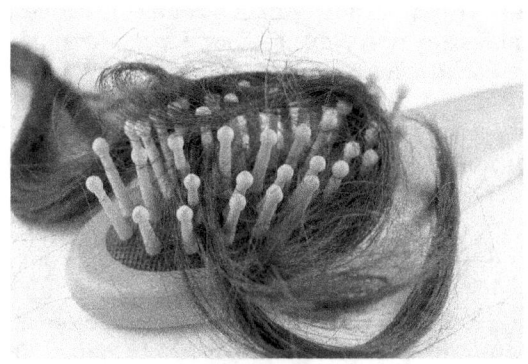

Photo by wong szefei

When the cocktail nurse first told me that I would surely lose my hair I winced. The thought of a fat, bald woman was a bad enough visual. The thought of the fat, bald woman being *me* was even worse. Already having self image issues, accepting myself as bald would be a hard sell. It's not that I have anything against bald people! My son is bald by choice and looks pretty good that way. Resigning to the "chrome dome" myself, however, is something else again! I decided I should take evasive action quickly!

I made an appointment with my hairdresser before even starting the chemo and had her cut my hair quite short. I decided that watching my longer hair fall out in clumps would be too traumatic. When she finished, I rather liked my hairstyle. Based on the compliments I received, apparently others did too. It's too bad the new "do" would be so short-lived. Together we developed a plan that when too much hair came out, we would give me a buzz.

I was warned by many that the hair would probably be out within 3 weeks of chemo. There were a few condescending folks that reassured me that my hair might only get thinner. That's where I am today, two weeks past the first chemo. The news flash is that "thinner" isn't much better than bald, and I think it is *time*. Although the loss is more subtle than I had expected, each time I wash my hair it seems to get shorter.

I should have never brought that second mirror into the bathroom. I should have never bent my head so that I could see the top of my head in the reflection! I was aghast! While I technically still have hair, I'm not so sure I want anyone to see it. Or perhaps it would be better stated that I don't want folks to see the fleshy scalp that keeps peeking boldly from beneath it! What's with this tender scalp stuff? Nobody mentioned *that*! Suddenly, scratching my head thoughtfully has transformed into an irritating habit that hurts!

Last night I went to Wal-Mart and bought a couple of scarves. I wasn't sure if you could buy scarves anymore, but the good Lord graced me with a healthy selection. I have a friend that works in that department and we laughed as I fumbled with all this material, twisting and tucking as I attempted to arrange it so that it would appear to be more attractive than a pile of cow poop sitting on my head. I was not successful at the store, but I bought the scarves anyway.

Google is my friend. Once home, I positioned myself in front of my keyboard, and started searching for instructions on how to wad this material on my head in a way that resembled something flattering. Although I finally succeeded in coming up with something similar to a turban, it took too long (no patience, remember), made me feel like a balloon in the Macy's parade , and it's heavy! I must admit that skullcaps, flattering or not on my fat face, are quick, lightweight, and cooler! Looking like a balloon face is preferable than looking like Mr. Clean, so I'll wear the skullcaps and scarves. The first person that offers me a string to keep me from floating away is going to get socked!

I must resign myself to the understanding that I have a poor self image, and even the most beautiful hat in the world would likely fall short of what I would see as flattering on myself. It's not the hat or scarf that is lacking here, but rather my confidence to feel comfortable in my own skin. So now you remind me that I purchased a wig. Yes I did. But the wig can't be tweaked until all of the hair is gone. Even though I know that it is probably time, I find myself procrastinating, and that is the real subject of this post.

What stops me from just shaving my head and getting it over with? Especially since I am not comfortable with my thin hair as it is? I find my procrastination a bit perplexing, so as usual for me, I begin to analyze it.

Women's hair has been an issue almost since the beginning of time. In cartoons like BC on the Rocks we depict cavemen dragging their women by it. Archaeological artifacts confirm that the women of Corinth wore both long and short hair. In the 1940's, women bobbed and permed it. The bible speaks of it often. Hair has been as much a part of our societal history as anything ever was or is. Men fantasize about women with long hair. From birth, women are taught, even if indirectly, that their hair is a crowning glory of sorts, that we have braided, twisted, bobbed, and manicured repeatedly during our waking moments since the dawn of civilization.

Cancer: It's Hair Raising!

Perhaps I feel like I'm bucking an age-old tradition, passed down through the generations. Maybe it's because I know my husband prefers me in long hair. Maybe having no hair is just too unfamiliar to be comfortable. Dwelling on the reasoning has not produced any fruitful conclusions that explain my bottom line: I just don't like it!

It's reasonable to me that I am plagued with a disease that provides a plethora of strange and unfamiliar side effects and issues, so it's not so hard to understand that I would cling to the familiar and predictable things in my life. My hair has always been a staple. Over the years it has been subjected to a variety of colors including purple, but it was still mine and it was still there. It is an issue that I have dealt with every morning when I start my day. It has been an accessory for my finest formalwear. It has been curled, straightened, cut, combed and coiffed. I know it inside and out, whether I like it or not. I am familiar with it.

Like everything else in my life these days, it is changing and this is a lot of change to deal with at my age. I have never shunned the unfamiliar, but the older I get, the less I embrace it. Familiar is to aging what comfort is to food. With each advancing year, I become more a creature of habit. That is, until cancer came along and turned my world upside down! I have a death grip on those things that remain comfortingly familiar and I am unwilling to give them up. I guess that my hair is one of those familiar comforts that is now being ripped from my grasp.

Thus, like two women fighting over a sale item, I am locked into a tug of war with my dragon over my hair. She yanks one way and I wrestle it back the other way. She's winning this particular battle. When I wear the cow poop scarf on my head, she rolls on the floor laughing, while my cheeks burn with embarrassment. Boy, she is annoying!

But sometimes we have to lose the battle in order to win the war. The fight over my hair is one she will win as I surrender my crown of glory one strand at a time, but I will strive to limit her victories and I will position myself for the next round on Tuesday, when I submit myself to the next cocktail. I guess my lack of hair will give her one less thing to grab onto when we tussle in that ring.

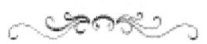

Cancer: The Trauma-Thursday, July 16, 2009

Last night my dragon had me on the ropes again and I was taking quite a beating. My hair had thinned so much that although I still had it, I was unwilling to allow others to see how spotty it had become. I knew that losing all my hair would be traumatic for me, but I underestimated how much.

Yesterday I went to Maurice's, a local clothing store with a 75% off sale. They sold scarves there and I thought that maybe a bright color would help cheer me up. While I was there, I tried on a couple tops that hugged a little more of me than I was comfortable with. Obviously, to get the top on and off, the scarf I was wearing became an impediment.

Wearing a wadded up scarf does nothing for the little bit of hairstyle I still possessed, so the unveiling presented a helter-skelter mess of what little bit was still there. While the locked dressing room provided concealment from others in the store, it did nothing to shelter me from the image that stared back at me in the mirror. Close to tears, I sadly exited the store with one garment and two scarves as I headed home to hide.

My emotions were already on the edge when 'Mas called from Wal-Mart, and our poor phone connection generated a frustrating and futile attempt to exchange information. Now I can add cranky to that list of emotional baggage I was toting. When 'Mas got home and asked me what was going on, I began to cry. My self esteem had hit a new low and I was ready to become a hermit because of it. My depression was, once again, on the rise.

After supper we watched a little television which distracted me some, but not enough. I seemed to be locked in this funk, like a ship struggling to find the shoreline in a dense fog. My smile had been exiled, my confidence on vacation as I curled up with a pillow into a ball on the couch. I felt so small.

'Mas suggested that even though the dragon would win this round, perhaps I should lessen her victory by taking control of how and when it happened. His idea made sense, although I was not at all sure I could do this and I couldn't cry continuously either. I mixed myself a couple of bloody marys while I mulled it over in my mind. I was hoping that the glass contained an ounce of courage among the vodka and the olives. A lorazepam chaser helped to dry my tears momentarily while I retrieved a chair from the kitchen.

Afternoons with Ivy

My dragon was standing in the corner of the room, smiling with anticipation. Her confidence was staggering. She strutted over to stand behind the chair. I needed 'Mas to be the barber because he was the one person I trusted most, and I knew that he would be protective of my feelings. This was going to be much harder than I thought.

I took my place in the chair and shuddered as 'Mas gathered the necessary tools. Before we began we prayed for God to get us through this latest crisis. As 'Mas put the blade to my forehead, sweeping it through what was left of my hair like a lawnmower blazes a path through a yard, I dissolved into hysterical wails. I knew that the initial strip of exposed flesh meant there was no turning back now and the finality of the effort wracked me with uncontrollable sobs.

Words cannot express how violated and vulnerable I felt. My dignity dissolved a little more with each stroke of the clipper. It seemed to take forever and I wondered when this torture would finally end. When at long last the final strand of hair hit the floor and the clipper grew silent, I was afraid to exhale. 'Mas lovingly brushed the hair from my shoulders and quickly removed the evidence that had collected on the floor. I grabbed a knitted cap that I knew had been made with loving hands and covered what I believed was my nakedness and my shame. By this time, my face was swollen like a basketball from all the tears and all I wanted was a dark place to hide.

I was so ashamed of what my appearance must be. I didn't want to see myself without hair. I wore that cap to the hot tub as well as to bed. Usually mornings bring with them a renewed sense of strength as well as a better outlook, but not today. I'm still not ready to stand in front of a mirror without a head cover. I'm still not ready to face the public. I am withdrawn, choosing to remain isolated, until I can get some sort of grip on this latest desecration of my former self.

My dragon is gloating. She is amused as we both study my reflection in the mirror. She baits me about removing my headpiece, but I won't yet. I feel defeated, violated and ugly. I am nearly choking on all this negativity. Yesterday was not a good day. Today may not be much better. I know that I will eventually adjust to this, but I underestimated how difficult this would be. For now, I need to pull back into the shadows and bask in my aloneness. Maybe tomorrow I will feel differently.

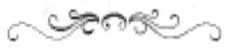

Cancer: God Bless Hairdressers!-

Thursday, July 16, 2009

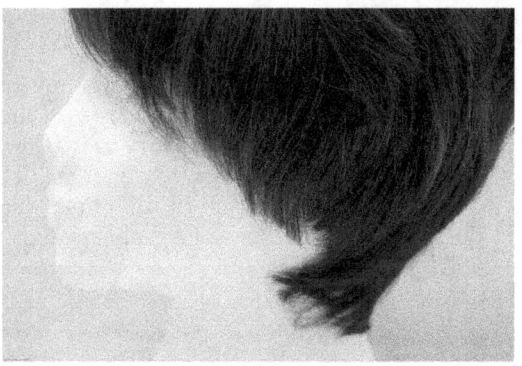

Photo by ilene swickle

God Bless hairdressers! At least God bless MY hairdresser. And praise God for wigs!

This morning I was still pretty blue and unwilling to face the public. But my hairdresser, Darla, who must be the most wonderful hairdresser ever, made a special effort to get me in tonight after her shop closed. I had purchased a wig before my chemo started, but it couldn't be fitted until my hair was gone and tonight was the night.

As I settled into the chair, Darla walked over and locked the door. 'Mas came along for moral support and took his position in a chair across from me. I asked if she needed to remove the wig, and requested that she turn the chair first so that I would not be facing the mirror. I still have not looked at myself without hair and that's just fine with me. I'm not ready to see myself without benefit of head covering. As Darla tweaked the wig, I would look nervously at 'Mas for his approval. It was always there.

It is wonderful to have hair on my head again, even if it isn't mine. In some ways it manages to do what I couldn't get my own hair to do. I've even decided I like the cap *with* the hair and I have uploaded some photos that 'Mas took so that you can see for yourself.

I can't wear the wig in the hot tub, and sleeping in it is a bad idea, but that is where Carol's nifty caps come in once again. Although the wig is clearly different than my own hairstyle, it looks reasonably natural, all things considered. Besides that, the wig makes it possible for me to almost totally ignore the fact that I have no hair of my own. Cleopatra is not the only one that can live by Denial!

My dragon is sulking because I didn't suffer enough. In my opinion I suffered *plenty*. Maybe 'Mas is correct, and choosing to shave off the pitiful small amount of hair that I had left mitigated her victory as it gave me back some control. Good! As it is, she got a much bigger chunk of me than I wanted her to have. She will no doubt live to harass me another day. Meanwhile, the next time I spar in the ring with her, when she grabs my hair, it will come off in her hand, and I will have the last laugh!

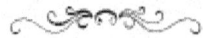

The block of granite

which was an obstacle in the pathway of the weak,

became a stepping-stone in the pathway of the strong.

~Thomas Carlyle

Cancer: Horizontal vs. Vertical-
Saturday, July 25, 2009

When broken down into its most basic form, chemotherapy can be divided into two simple categories-- Horizontal and vertical. I'm either up and moving around, or I am flattened and probably asleep. Now that I have had my second cocktail, I'm noticing that I spend more time in the latter state than in the former.

There have been a few other changes as well that have not gone unnoticed. The shot given to stimulate the bone marrow comes with an assortment of aches and pains similar to aging on steroids. Lucky for me we have a hot tub that allows me to submerse my sore back and achy knees. I figure if I can't cure what ails me, maybe I can drown it!

I have finally accepted my baldness, although I don't hang out with mirrors and reserve my exhibitionism to those who visit me within the confines of my own safe sanctuary. When I do go out, I still modestly cover what is left of my former crowning glory with some semblance of protection. These days my head resembles a fuzzy peach rather than a head of hair and I look like an elf with pointy-looking ears. The cocktails make my scalp sore, and I have tried a variety of topical concoctions in an effort to soothe the itchy, burning sensation that the cocktail creates. I think that today I have finally found my solution with an aloe-vera product mixed with lidocaine and intended to relieve sunburn. Since it's been sitting in my bathroom closet for nearly ten years, I'm thinking I'd better use it sparingly! Replacing it may be more difficult than I think!

I have encountered my first experience with scent sensitivity that I was forewarned of. There are just some smells that turn the stomach during chemo week, although that is the extent of the nausea I have experienced. The stomach cramps remain an issue, but fortunately I have been taking the prilosec since the first cocktail, so the ongoing treatment dissuades too much discomfort. This is not a dietary method that I would endorse, but my appetite is a mere a shadow of its former self, and I have lost about eight pounds. Sadly, those pounds are an insignificant representation of what I need to lose overall, so my weight loss is not all that impressive.

I guess I mention all this for that person that next follows in my footsteps. Although chemotherapy isn't a pleasant experience, it could be much worse, and it is certainly doable. Any woman who has ever been pregnant is familiar with the horror stories so graciously shared by others who have gone before. Chemotherapy isn't much different. In my experience, however, the fear factor is highly overrated and the horror stories that you do hear probably won't be coming from other cancer survivors. While unpleasant, it doesn't warrant the fear that I gave it initially. My advice after two cocktails is use a port, and expect lots of horizontal days the week of your chemo treatments. By the end of the second week and through most of the third week following your cocktail, you are going to feel more normal than not.

There is no doubt in my mind that to date, the greatest trauma has been centered around the hair, or loss of it. Without a doubt, that has become the toughest hurdle so far. In buzzing the hair off, I thought that I could maintain some control over my dragon, thus minimizing her impact. In hindsight I'm not at all certain that this is true and if I were to do it again, I'm not sure I would choose the buzz over letting the short hair fall out on its own.

I am convinced that cancer is a very individual experience, and there is no art or science to coping through it. What works for one may not work for another and the ability to cope is very much influenced by each individual's life experiences. Without benefit of those specific life experiences, judgment of how an individual chooses to live or die with cancer should be best left unspoken. Attention needs to be directed to how one can be more supportive rather than more judgmental. I would invite anyone who has never lived through cancer to step to the front of the line, setting the bar by example, but I would be surprised if there were any takers and as long as there are no takers, neither is there any room to assume how cancer should be done correctly.

Having said this, my dragon leans over my shoulder, snorting smoke as if to say that the battle rages between us exclusive to outsiders. We each harbor our own dragons, and must devise our own methods of slaying them.

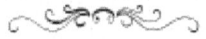

I may have spoken a bit prematurely since yesterday I was, once again, trading fisticuffs with my dragon. She is certainly as persistent as a pimple during a period and even less welcome!

I have coined a new phrase for the side effects that accompany the chemo cocktails over time which I have christened "cocktail buildup". With each round of cocktail served, a certain amount of chemo remains in my system, overlapping with the next round and generating a buildup of toxins. Although these effects follow a basic pattern of sorts, my dragon ducks and weaves, taking advantage of her element of surprise by adding modifications to our usual ringside dance.

Just when I think I am finally vertical, a swift swish of her tail knocks me horizontal once again. A quick kick to my groin renews the stomach cramps. She rakes her talons over my scalp only to leave her mark with a searing discomfort. At this point I'm left to wonder, "Who's on first?" I don't think it is me. Like the classic comedy routine performed by Abbott and Costello, cancer and chemotherapy are muddled with confusion and doubletalk. My dragon, like Abbott, works hard to keep me confused, uninformed, and confounded, despite my best efforts to remain educated.

My oncologist warns me of the dangers of fever while assuring me that he is only a phone call away irrespective of time and date. Twice I have availed his service with questions about side effects, and twice I have been left to my own devices and common sense. My dragon is rolling her eyes and chuckling as if to say, "Did you really believe they would be there for you?" I hope I'm not paying for those phone calls! As the doctor on call explained that he couldn't see the rash unless I went to the office, and the office is closed because it is Sunday, I rolled my eyes and considered calling Guido and his boys to give the doc a lesson in compassion! I decided to take some benadryl which seems to have helped considerably. I logic out that I am having a reaction to one of the drugs, but have no way of determining which one. *That* is part of the expertise that I *thought* my insurance premiums were buying.

I had requested a pet scan at the end of chemo in the hopes of gleaning some peace of mind that we have at least killed this dragon before another one presents herself. For reasons I don't yet understand, my oncologist has communicated that he doesn't favor such a test, and states that I may never know if the chemo worked or not.

"How will I know then?" I asked. Each cocktail costs $10K, so expecting to know if I have a clean baseline to start the next potential bout with seems reasonable enough to me. "By your symptoms," he responds indelicately. "But I didn't have any symptoms until I had a golf ball sized tumor in my breast!" I was thinking of something a bit more proactive! When questioned about how they plan to monitor my body for further breakouts, the oncologist assured me that I would have mammograms done every 6 months and I would be on medication for the next few years. This might sound good in theory, but my surgeon told me that he would stop just short of diagnosing me as a stage 4 because although the cancer had metastasized in my lymph nodes and was likely traveling, he couldn't say where it was likely to be.

Now I am wondering how a semi-annual mammogram will tell anyone if the cancer has relocated itself in my brain or my bones. When I press the oncologist for the answer to that question, he insists that we will continue the discussion at the end of chemotherapy which translates in my brain to "I don't know", ...third base. My dragon watches this interchange with amusement. She knows that a lack of honest communication between me and my doctors tips the odds in her favor. I know it too. So how come this college graduate doesn't get that?

"What about all those other folks in remission? How do they know that?," I challenge. He informs me that unless they are cancer free for ten years they do NOT know that, and their proclamations amount to wishful thinking. Well that's encouraging, NOT. Our meeting ends in a stalemate. Eyes locked in conflict, nobody blinks except my dragon, who claps her hands with glee at the teamwork spelled with so many I's.

So to date my interactions with the oncologist keep me spinning in circles! What happens when I get to second base? That depends on who's on first base, me or my dragon. As yet, I don't know...third base.

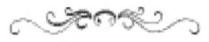

Cancer: Courage of the Heart-

Tuesday, July 28, 2009

Some days my focus is limited to renewing my strength and courage. Today seems to be one of those days. I'm always searching for new input that keeps the battle in perspective. It makes sense to me that others struggle with their own dragons and although their dragons are different than mine, they are no less exhausting. With that in mind, today my thoughts are on those countless others who might feel strengthened and renewed by the encouragement I have sought out. To those people, this one is for you. Pause and be refreshed.

Yesterday I dared to struggle. Today I dare to win. ~ Bernadette Devlin

The best way out is always through. ~ Robert Frost

Feed your faith and your fears will starve to death. ~Author Unknown

Some days there won't be a song in your heart. Sing anyway. ~Emory Austin

Turn your face to the sun and the shadows fall behind you. ~Maori Proverb

Courage is being afraid but going on anyhow. ~Dan Rather

When you come to the end of your rope, tie a knot and hang on. ~Franklin D. Roosevelt

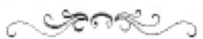

Afternoons with Ivy

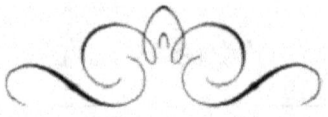

Lyrics from "Tough"

by Craig Morgan

...We sat there five years ago

The doctors let us know

She'd have to fight to live, I broke down and cried

She held me and said it's gonna be alright

She wore that wig to church

Pink ribbon pinned there on her shirt

No room for fear, full of faith

Hands held high singing Amazing Grace

Never once complained, refusing to give up

And I thought I was tough...

Lyrics to "Just Stand Up"

by Various Artists

The heart is stronger Than you think, It's like it can go through anything
And even when you think It can't it finds a way to still push on, though
Sometimes you want to run away, Ain't got the patience For the pain
And if you don't believe it look into your heart, The beat goes on
I'm tellin' you Things get better through whatever
If you fall dust it off don't let up
Don't you know you can go be your own miracle
You need to know

CHORUS
If the mind keeps thinking you've had enough
But the heart keeps telling you don't give up
Who are we to be Questioning & Wondering what is what
Don't give up. Through it all just stand up

It's like We all have better days, problems getting all up in your face
Just because you go through it don't mean it got to take control, no
You ain't gotta find no hiding place because the heart can beat the hate
Don't wanna let your mind Keep playin' you and sayin' you can't go on
Things get better through whatever
If you fall dust it off don't let up
Don't you know you can go be your own miracle
You need to know

CHORUS

You don't gotta be A prisoner in your mind
If you fall dust it off
You can live your life, yeah
Let your heart be your guide, Yeah, yeah, yeah
And you will know that you're good if you trust in the good
Everything will be alright, yeah
Light up the dark If you follow your heart and it will get better through
whatever

CHORUS

You got it in you, Find it within, You got in now, Find it within now
You got in you, Find it within, You got in now, Find it within now
THROUGH IT ALL, JUST STAND UP!

Cancer: Silver Linings?-

I firmly believe that behind every dark cancer cloud is a silver lining, although sometimes they are harder to see than at other times. A good friend once suggested that, during those harder times, making a list of blessings can provide a good distraction, while it reinforces positive thinking.

Yesterday I decided to give my friend's idea a try and make a list of blessings that I have received because of cancer. It's not a long list, but there are a few things that I can be thankful for, at least temporarily.

Blessing #1: *I never have a bad hair day.* When God gave me hair, he skimped a bit on the thick, luxurious locks that adorn the heads of so many others. Instead I got thin, limp hair that has just enough natural wave to fall awkwardly around my shoulders. Each morning my clothes, mood, and confidence are determined by how my hair is behaving. To insure the best outcome, I wash my hair daily so that it will better cooperate. Since cancer, and the complete absence of my hair, this whole exercise becomes a moot issue! When you have no hair at all, you can't sleep on it wrong! Rumor has it that my hair will grow back thick and curly. While I'm not sure that I'm crazy about the curly part, I'm looking forward to the thickness, and will be disappointed if it remains just a rumor.

Blessing #2: *Through the course of the chemo treatments, I will not have to shave the hair on my legs and armpits.* Aren't you jealous? I know that I am not the only woman who appreciates winter and long pants because they hide our laziness about shaving our legs! For the first time in my post-pubescent life I am not concerned with razor stubble! My legs are as smooth as a baby's bottom!

Blessing #3: *Along these same lines, I am no longer plagued with that persistent chin hair!* Hallelujah! In my opinion, women were not designed to grow beards, so when my 55th birthday ushered in embarrassing chin hairs, I was none too happy! Amazingly, the hair on my head takes years to acquire any length, but the hairs on my chin sprout like weeds after a rainstorm! With diminished eyesight, plucking became impractical. The luxury of a salon waxing worked for awhile, until the hair grew so quickly that the $8 treatment turned into a $40 weekly expense! That is an unacceptable pocket shock for a frugal person like me!

I figured that I could smear hot wax on my chin as easily as anyone else. WRONG! Someone needs to develop a timer on those wax heaters to prevent the wax from reaching 1000 degrees Fahrenheit! I'm here to testify that the scabbing burns on a scalded chin draw far more attention than those little hairs ever could! Add to that the necessity of explaining why you have scabs on your chin which adds even more humiliation! I bought a lumineeze. Have you tried that one yet? It just yanks those little hairs out by the roots. My chin is tough and can take it, but my upper lip will have none of this! So at least for the time being, chemo has eliminated a very frustrating problem for me.

Blessing #4: *Thanks to chemo, most foods have very little, if any, taste* so I am not as apt to binge. I may always be a carb junkie, but when decadent chocolates and green salads start tasting the same, there ceases to be an incentive for hiding in the bathroom to inhale a candy bar out of sight of potentially judgmental eyes. And if the lack of taste isn't motivating enough, the mouth sores will certainly convince anyone to skip a meal!

Blessing #5: *Chemo offers the opportunity to develop new hobbies with new friends.* I have taken up pole-dancing! I have developed an intimate relationship at my oncologist's office with a gal named Ivy (I.V.). I see her with each visit to the cocktail lounge, she goes everywhere I go, and she never leaves my side. She's tall, skinny and chrome. Our relationship is not without its hangups, and I mean that quite literally! Ivy is attached to me via a maze of tubes, and like two awkward dancers, we are often entangled and tripping over each other. Since I never get a moment away from Ivy, she also becomes a bit suffocating. Friends are nice, but no one wants to spend all of their time with them!

Blessing #6: Aging has been a struggle that I do not do gracefully and memory has long been a casualty of that process. I often complain that I have the memory of a gnat. With chemotherapy, this problem becomes compounded by "chemo brain". The bad news is that I will probably forget that we had planned to do lunch together. *The good news is that you can vent anything to me without fear of reprisal because I will forget it within a half hour of hearing it!* Chemo brain also makes for a handy explanation of why I am late, why I forgot, or how come I failed to do something that I told you I would do. I am no longer reliable for remembered tasks, so you should expect this.

Blessing #7: I have never had the patience to be a sun goddess. My job keeps me glued to a desk chair by a computer, and fluorescent lights keep me a healthy pasty white. Since tan is "in", I'm usually noticeably "out". Any tan that I manage to acquire comes only through activities that coincidentally happen outdoors and not because I soak up the rays intentionally. *Thanks to chemo, I have finally acquired a legitimate reason for remaining several shades lighter than most* and no longer have to concern myself with explanations of why I resemble a mushroom that lives in the dark instead of sporting a glowing, bronze sheen. I can flash my wrinkle-free smile that matches the whiteness of my teeth without guilt or shame.

Now that I have made my list of blessings, I do feel better about my cancer-ridden body, especially that chin thing! I have adequately distracted myself from the stomach cramps (praise God for imodium), my sore, itchy scalp and my incredible fatigue. Gee, I feel SO much better!

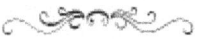

Cancer is a word, not a sentence.

~John Diamond

Cancer: Over the Hump?-Monday, August 17, 2009

When chemo first started, I wore 6 bracelets on my left arm, each representing a week of chemotherapy. As each chemo session arduously passed, I would remove one bracelet and know at a glance how many were left. Each bracelet symbolized a journey through these unchartered waters called cancer and the remaining bracelets became symbolic of a hope for an end in sight.

This past week I completed the half way mark. Like the proverbial "over the hump" Wednesday, I am half way home, yet I am left to consider just what that means or if it means anything at all. While each of the chemo weeks bear some similarities, they remain individual in the myriad of small ways that this poison invades my body. I have to remind myself that there is a point to all of this and that tolerating the next time has a purpose. For the benefit of those souls who follow my bread crumbs along this path I walk, I think that I am finally experienced enough to provide a glimpse of what to expect as well as how to cope with it, although admittedly I am less adequate in the latter than I care to admit.

I guess that it would be pertinent here to point out that the side effects will vary depending on the cocktail of choice. My cocktail has been chosen to be kinder to my existing heart condition, and while it reduces my survival rate from 80% to 50%, the side effects I experience are also kinder, so I am aware that things could be much worse.

This particular half way point was not without a few earmarks of its own. My week actually started on Monday with a trip to an endocrinologist and the hope of stabilizing my blood sugar which has been an ongoing battle from the get-go. By adding insulin injections to my daily regime it is my hope that I can better protect my failing vision. The steroids administered in the chemo process are very upsetting to that delicate balance, typically skyrocketing my blood sugars into the 600+ ranges instead of the 100 range that they should be. The oncologist has been forced to cut both the IV and oral version of steroids drastically. As I understand it, one of the purposes of the steroid is to protect my already compromised liver from the taxotere cocktail which is extremely debilitating to it. By drawing my own blood four times a day, and then injecting a mathematically determined insulin chaser, the hope is that I can eventually receive the steroid necessary to protect my already ailing liver.

This chemo week officially began on Tuesday, as it always does. Like all chemo weeks, I have to be driven to the cocktail lounge by someone else because I am given a certain amount of sedation throughout the course of the cocktail. I go to the QC for my chemo, so there is a 2 hour round-trip commute involved in the process. Once there, my first order of business is to weigh in. Stepping on a scale has never been something I look forward to, but even with the inclusion of steroids that are known to add pounds I continue to show a weight loss, albeit minimal. Next is a blood draw to determine if my platelets are adequate enough to get me through the upcoming chemo process. From there I meet with the oncologist to discuss side effects and the measures for minimizing them. Most recently, they have added antibiotics to combat the angry rash on my scalp, and Imodium for the ongoing intestinal problems. The mouth sores and pain in my feet are temporary side effects that come and go on their own. After that I proceed to the cocktail lounge where I spend the next four hours with Ivy, pumping the needed poisons into my system. Although I am exhausted by the end of that day, the real fatigue doesn't hit me until later.

Each Wednesday of chemo week I need another ride back to the QC for a follow up shot of neulasta, intended to kick my bone marrow into high gear. It does that, but it also gives me flu symptoms for the next three or four days, makes my muscles and joints ache and runs up a fever of 101.3. This last time I arranged to bring the shot home with me so that 'Mas can inject me, hopefully sparing me the exhausting trip back to the QC and eliminating the need to locate a driver to shuttle me back and forth. As has been the case up to this point, the Wednesday trip totally wipes me out, and it is not uncommon for me to be asleep shortly after I get home until Friday morning with little, if any, waking time. I'm not supposed to harbor a fever due to my reduced immunity level, so the first order of business is to minimize the fever to no more than 100.5. The fever will come and go for days later, and my energy level cannot sustain much more than 15 minutes at a time. As I write this, I am still fighting the roller coaster of body temperature that takes its toll on me.

Again, this last chemo brought its own set of variations. I have a medical port beneath the skin of my neck for inserting the chemo and taking blood draws. The idea is to spare my veins from collapsing after repeated use, but the port is no longer functioning exactly as it should. Drawing blood from the port has been unsuccessful and injecting the chemical cocktail has been slowed to a snail's crawl. There is a small amount of discomfort as the poisons are pumped in through the port, so it was decided to inject a clot buster into the port in an effort to see if there is some sort of clot blockage. When that effort returned no answers, it was decided that a dye needed to be injected to insure that there wasn't a kink in the port. This is done in a hospital environment, so the needle was left in, I was given the cocktail through a standard vein, and another appointment for the dye test was added to the following day's trip in for the neulasta shot. In the event of a kink, the port would need to be surgically modified if it is to be serviceable, so I was glad that no blockage was found. It was determined that the problem was the result of a fibrin sheath that allows the injection of the chemicals, albeit more slowly, but does not allow for the blood draw. I was relieved to hear that I could continue using the port for the cocktail, but disappointed to learn that blood draws would have to be done in a more traditional method. By the end of Wednesday, my energy level was fully spent, and I was down for the count. I didn't really wake again until Friday morning and because of the neulasta, I experienced the flu-like symptoms through the weekend.

Typically throughout chemo week I am home alone during the day. For the first two days I am mostly asleep, so am unaware of my surroundings as well as my aloneness. By the end of the week, however, I am awake enough to realize my solitude but not enough to justify a request for companionship that I am unlikely to have the energy to sustain. While on one hand I am very lonely and depressed, I am also too tired and ill to appreciate company. TGIF! By the end of work week, 'Mas comes home for the weekend and I am comforted by his presence. This past weekend, we spent a large percentage of time with me curled up in bed grateful for 'Mas' arms around me. Usually, the side effects of the chemo interfere with my ability to get to church on that Sunday and this week was no exception. I feel too weak and ill to deal with life outside my bedroom.

Because of a conversation with my oncologist, I have been fighting even more emotional issues that the anti-depressant isn't overcoming. When I asked my oncologist how we would know that the last chemo cocktail had killed all of the existing cancer, he responded that we may never know. What if the chemo was too gentle for the aggressive type of cancer that they say I have? What if all of it doesn't die? What if I have endured all these side effects for naught? Are we really curing me or just watching me die more slowly? Sometimes those questions overwhelm me. Sometimes I grieve for my life back as I knew it before. There is so much cancer around me that at times it chokes me with its stench. I feel so trapped! My dragon becomes a constant companion and eerily, I am getting used to her presence. Like Stockholm Syndrome, she is becoming a familiar entity in an unfamiliar world.

Sometimes, like now, all I can do is cry. Cry for what was, for what could have been, and for what might never be. I know God is with me, but what if this is how He plans for me to end? Will it hurt? They have told me that my cancer is likely to return. Will I survive this time only to have to do it all again? Where am I going and what is going to happen to me? Until mortality slaps you in the face like this, knowing something and living it are two very different things. A crisis of faith seems natural.

Afternoons with Ivy

We went to the relay for life. I have gone each year since Heidi died to witness the lighting of her luminary. This year was very different. We arrived at dusk, and took a walk around the lake. It was very hot, and although I wore my wig, my head was roasting. I found a bench to wait for the lighting ceremony and as the dark night sky replaced the sun, I dared to remove the wig and allow my head to breath. There was a certain safety with the darkness. I determined that here, of all places, I should be safe. My dragon whispers that there are no other bald people present, which made my comfort tentative at best. The ceremony started with a reading of a poem about a "dark room". Although the poem bothered me, I managed to sit through it. Next came a song sung by a care-giver about the loss of a loved one. That one did me in. I announced that I needed to go, and quickly darted through the crowd like a shot, gratefully exiting the park in record time. This year the ceremony took on a very different flavor, and it was just too close for comfort. Part of me felt disloyal to Heidi. I had been there for her in the past. This time I could not be, which made me feel sad.

I know that self pity is never a good thing, but at times, it becomes unavoidable. At times I want to scream at something, anything that will allow me to vent my rage. I want to beat my fists on the chest of this dragon and kick my way out of this abyss that I seem to have fallen in. I feel as though I am spiraling out of control, like a plane spinning recklessly towards the earth, destined to burst into flames upon impact.

By the end of the second week after chemo week, some normalcy returns to my life. I manage to put a tentative lid on my panic and fear. I force back the stench and smoke of my dragon whose presence lingers ever next to me. I open a window to suck out the smoke that her nostrils evoke so that I can breathe. I look away from her piercing yellow eyes, redirecting my focus as best that I can just in time to do it all again. Each chemo week lasts longer, and overcoming the demons becomes more difficult. There are more of them to vanquish and I have less strength to fight them with. Even the end of chemo is not the end of the cancer. There remains more surgery and radiation, ongoing mammograms and blood workups. Certainly life as I knew it will never be again.

I think about retiring at 62. I learned at tax school that if you expect a shorter life span, you should opt out at 62, The reality is that I might never see 62, even though it remains a mere four years away because I am told that my cancer is likely to reappear within three years. The plans that 'Mas and I made for our golden years may never see fruition and the tears begin again. There are just too many tears and I am running out of places to put them.

To that soul following my bread crumb trail, you will need a large vessel for all those tears. Like your dragon, they will follow you for the rest of your life, however long that might be.

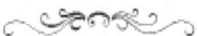

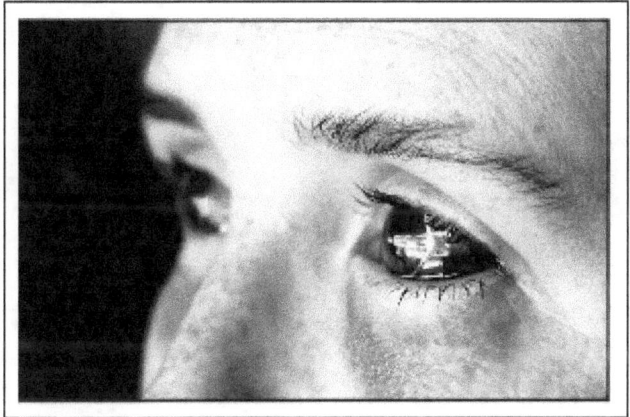

Photo by Stephanie Swartz

Even in my bleakest moments, when my muscles ache, my scalp burns like fire, my cramps bend me into a ball and I'm so weak that I dare not move even a heartbeat from my bed, the loving support of friends and family get me through. In my darkest moments the one truth I never question is that God has blessed me richly with the love of others who are willing to go the extra mile on my behalf and I am so grateful for them.

Whoever you are, if you are reading this blog, there is a strong likelihood that you are among those loyal and steadfast individuals who have served us meals each week, transported me to chemotherapy and back again for those questionably "helpful" shots, pulled my weeds, concerned yourself with my comforts, prayed for me, sent me light, emailed me encouragement or spent the postage to send me a card. I get lost in the list of ways that so many have done so much for us.

I have received more encouraging books than I will ever live long enough to read. I wear bracelets proclaiming what cancer cannot do to me, and key chains of pink ribbons that contain the keys to the world of my existence. I have a plaque on one of my walls that reminds me of God's shroud of protection over my head. And speaking of heads, I wear hats that cover my nakedness, knitted by loving hands and scarves that declare my uniqueness known only to those who have cared to learn what that uniqueness is. Each and every gift represents the love that you send and that I receive. Some of you even manage to pull a smile to my lips when I need it most, drying the tears in my eyes, at least temporarily.

What I am wanting to convey here is that in whatever way you have opened your hearts to 'Mas and I, you should know that it has touched us deeply, and often has been the much needed lift that chases away my dragon, even if only for a moment. For that, you have earned our undying admiration and appreciation. I will walk through fire for you as long as I draw breath to walk. There is little that you would ask of me that I would not attempt to accomplish for you, even though you are much too polite to ask.

Often, I am too ill to call you and thank you personally. I try to send a personal note but there are so many doing so much, that sometimes I just lose track of who I've contacted and who I've failed to contact. Chemo douses a fertile memory, which leaves me at a disadvantage. In spite of this, you must know that you make a difference in my struggling efforts to conquer this dragon, and I pray that is enough acknowledgement to encourage you to continue spreading love and hope to others whatever their plight in life might be. I read each guest book entry praying for blessings for each person who takes the time to pen a sentiment.

Perhaps that is the greatest lesson that I take from this God forsaken experience. It serves to soften the edges of what is otherwise a harsh and difficult experience, particularly during those chemo weeks. The lesson is that I am loved, albeit undeserved or unwarranted, and I thank God for that.

The Second lesson, which is no less important, is that I love you too. Even during those dark hours and lonely times, life goes on and so do your struggles, and though they be of a different nature than mine, they are no less significant or important. You are important to me, and your struggles are important to me too, even in the midst of my own. I pray for you daily, asking God to bless you for your compassion and kindness of heart. Which brings me to my second unquestionable truth...my knowledge that God rewards compassion and looks lovingly on a heart of mercy. I desire to share in your joys, mingle my tears with yours, and stand firmly at your side in your darkest hour, just as you have done for me. If it isn't God's will that I win this war, you must know that I will continue to stand on your behalf, wherever I am. There are some bonds that even death cannot break.

Kahlil Gibron, a favorite author of mine, wrote a book entitled "The Prophet" which has long held deep meaning for me. In the final chapter he speaks of death and God so eloquently, some quotes of which I would choose to share with you here:

"Let not the waves of the sea separate us now, and the years you have spent in our midst become a memory...only another breath will I breathe in this still air, only another loving look cast backward, and then I shall stand among you, a seafarer among seafarers."

Of Love he says, "Like sheaves of corn He gathers you unto Himself. He threshes you to make you naked. He sifts you to free you from your husks. He grinds you to whiteness. He kneads you until you are pliant; and then He assigns you to His sacred fire, that you may become sacred bread for God's sacred feast...When love beckons to you follow Him, though His ways are hard and steep. And when His wings enfold you yield to Him, though the sword hidden among His pinions may wound you...When you love you should not say 'God is in my heart,' but rather, 'I am in the heart of God'."

Of Pain, Gibron says, "And the cup He brings, though it burn your lips, has been fashioned of the clay which the Potter has moistened with His own sacred tears."

Gibron goes on to say, "Your fear of death is but a trembling of the Shepherd when He stands before the King whose hand is to be laid upon Him in honor. Is the Shepherd not joyful beneath His trembling, that He shall wear the mark of the King? Yet is He not more mindful of His trembling? For what is it to die but to stand naked in the wind and to melt into the sun? And what is it to cease breathing, but to free the breath from its restless tides, that it may rise and expand and seek God unencumbered? Only when you drink from the river of silence shall you indeed sing."

So much of what Gibron writes speaks to my heart and my faith. From his words I draw strength and comfort as they sing to me as a song, and what a sweet melody it is. My circumstances leave me no choice but to consider death. My faith permits me to look beyond death, which is too simple an answer to such a complex question as life. The words reassure me that no matter how dire my situation, I will prevail, be it in this life or another. Cancer cannot take that from me regardless of what else it strips.

It's never too soon to say "thank you" and never too late to profess love. While you encourage me with your compassion, I would encourage you to continue sharing your love no matter what the season. Someone is listening , needing to hear it and you say it so well. :^)

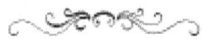

rec ·on ·cil ·i ·a ·tion–noun 1. an act of reconciling or the state of being reconciled. 2. the process of making consistent or compatible.

The diagnosis of cancer is a death sentence, and whether I beat it or whether I don't, there remains a process that must be undertaken to prepare me for whatever the outcome. I call that reconciliation. Reconciliation doesn't mean that I am giving up. It merely suggests that I need to find some compatibility with *all* of the possibilities. I don't want to die, nor do I intend to submit to this disease that threatens me without an incredible fight. But like it or not, win, lose or draw, we have no way of predicting God's will or His timing, and I must be at the ready.

When I speak of my potential death, it makes others uncomfortable. They awkwardly protest. What they don't understand is that just in case this is God's time for me, I need to have my house in order. I need to evaluate my life, mending fences, changing attitudes, forgiving wrongs, and making the best of the time that I have. I'm thinking this is something to embrace rather than turn away from. If I survive, how much better person will I have become? Win-win. To face death but do nothing to reconcile my life strikes me as just plain stupid and while I'm considered a little bit crazy, I'm not stupid.

If you are honest with yourself, how many times have you been too busy to reach out to someone you know needs you? How many times have you glossed over the opportunity to build memories because there is work to be done? We all do it. What does it take to get us to slow down and smell those roses? We lie to ourselves and tell ourselves that we'll do it tomorrow but tomorrow never seems to come and before we know it, tomorrow is too late. Sometimes we become so absorbed in our todays, that it takes an act of God to stop us long enough to consider our tomorrows   Everyone's life is a story. When we pause to consider why God allows such things in this life, perhaps we should also consider that without them we might miss the climax of our stories. There have been many times that God has spoken to me with that soft, still voice and I have either ignored it or failed to hear it due to the loud clamoring of my own voice. I have often joked about God's velvet 2x4. In my case at least, cancer was a swing of that velvet 2x4. I should clarify that I do not believe God gave me cancer, but I do believe that I was missing His message so He permitted me have it. It certainly got my attention! (Job 1:1-12)

The point is that, when faced with our mortality, we harbor an instinctive need to look at it. I don't speak of my own death to upset anyone. Nor do I mention it as a pathetic excuse to garner self pity. I am reconciling. I am asking myself the hard questions. I'm taking a critical examination of my own life, and insuring that I am ready. God may not take me today or tomorrow, but he will take me at some time and in some way. I will likely not get any advance notice of it. Therefore I must be at the ready. Being told that I am dying forces me to ask myself, "Am I ready?" in a serious way that my busyness would probably not take the time to consider. Developing the willingness to let go of the people and things that I love here is not a simple task. It becomes a process and like all processes, it requires thought and preparation.

Anyone that knows me also knows my penchant to overanalyze even the simplest of things. My Type A++ personality leaks into every cell of my being. Is it really so surprising that I would face something as important as my life, relationships and love without a microscope? For me that analysis often includes verbalizing what I see so that I can penetrate the storm in my own mind long enough to absorb it. So don't cringe when I mention my own demise. Understand that I am merely taking stock and making sure that I am ready. With God's will it won't be now.

If you could have an opportunity to say goodbye, would you take it? Based on my recent experiences, I think that you would. I know that I would. I want the people I love to know that they are loved, NOW and from my own lips. If I have a chance to right a wrong, I want to do it NOW. If there is an opportunity to forgive, let it be NOW. When I stand before God, (and I will stand before God), reviewing my life, I don't want to stare sheepishly at my toes while he asks me why I didn't say I was sorry, or why I didn't help, or why I turned away.

I'm not happy about having cancer. In biblical times I would be rending my robe in grief. I do not want to leave the people I love, even though I know that I will be going to another place far greater. I don't let go of love that easily. I'm betting that most don't. Death is not a simple, "oh, okay" response. It is a gut-wrenching peeling of the skin that contains us. Leaving will not be easy, and we all will leave. When you fillet a fish, the meat must be stripped from the bone and the skin peeled from the meat. I don't believe that saying goodbye to the ones that we love is any easier.

So to face death is to face reconciliation. Reconciliation is a responsibility, We have to insure that we are ready, for ourselves and for those that we leave behind. Most of us won't do it without some sort of prompting. We are too busy, or just too afraid. You don't plan a trip without packing for it. Eventually we are all going away. By the time this dragon of mine is slain, my bags will be packed, and when my ticket arrives, I will be ready to leave. But I will cast a backward glance, and there will be tears in my eyes. Are YOU ready? Just what will it take to get YOU that way?

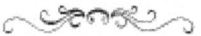

Ready to Fly by FFH

I've been grounded far too long
I'm ready to see the open wide
Ready to sing a different song
I've seen my troubles 'long the way
I want to sail towards the sun
I want to turn another page
I'm on my way

I'm ready to fly,
I'm ready to soar
I'm ready to leave this world behind.
I'm ready to open up the door
I'm ready to fly,
I'm ready to spread my wings across the sky
I think it's time
I'm ready to go
I'm ready to fly.

You've told me I could rise above
Like an eagle on the wind
I can glide upon Your love
But I feel the pull of gravity
And it's a weight upon my shoulders
I can't stay here any longer
I've gotta be free

And it's been so long
Since I've seen the bright morning sun
Through the early morning horizon
And it's been so long
Since I've felt the air under my wings
And seen all of these things from above

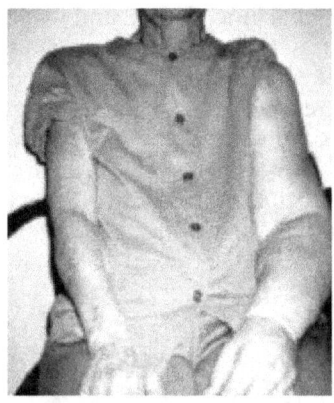

Does the left arm in the picture seem grotesque to you? It did to my mother as well, but her arm looked like this for twenty years because she had lymphedema that accelerated into elephantiasis when it went untreated. Now I have lymphedema. It results as a byproduct when lymph nodes are removed during breast cancer surgery and can be life threatening. This photo in conjunction with my mother's experience may help to explain my paranoia about getting lymphedema as well as my extreme reaction when I realized I had it. To make matters worse, its appearance may be a result of my own carelessness! There is no cure for lymphedema.

I have been SOOOO careful to avoid this problem. I wear a medical i.d. bracelet on my right arm warning all medical personnel off from blood pressure and blood draws which are known to bring it on. When we hot tub, my right arm is never immersed more than momentarily because hot water can cause it to flare. There are a myriad of things that can antagonize it, including ordinary bug bites. The mind boggles!

Friday morning started like any other morning. My first task of the day is to check my blood sugar level so that I can administer my first shot of insulin. Since my last chemo, I have been doing this four times a day every day. After two weeks of sticking and injecting, my fingertips had gotten a bit sore, so I opted to take my sample from my left arm. I didn't notice my dragon hovering closely behind me. It was a vertical week, so I had almost forgotten about her, but she hadn't forgotten me! As I pulled the trigger for the prick from my good arm, I got nothing. I didn't see her scaly finger cover the needle entry and block the blood flow. Without thinking I repeated the procedure in my right arm. The blood appeared quickly and I finished the process. Because the effort had gone so easily in my right arm, I instinctively used it again at lunch. It wasn't long after that my arm began to swell noticeably. My dragon must have been giddy with glee.

'Mas had called me during his lunch break, and while talking to him I noticed that the medical alert bracelet on my right arm, usually quite loose, had become tight. When I looked at my arm, I recognized the swelling, and my mind flashed back to my mother's arm when her lymphedema first started. I panicked! Rushing to the phone I dialed the surgeon's office and spoke with his nurse. What should I do??? She instructed me to wrap the arm with the materials she had given me the last time I saw her, and then elevate it as long as possible. I was devastated! Meanwhile, my dragon was dancing a jig. The understanding that I may well have caused this myself sent my heart plummeting and my head reeling.

I nervously crossed the street to my neighbor Mary Ann, armed with the bandages and tape. She helped me wrap my arm, and with it propped airborne over my head, I made my way back home to the safety of my bed where I sat that way for the next several hours. I don't mind saying that my arm got quite heavy and hard to hold up, but I was desperate! I prayed feverishly, begging God to reverse my mistake and swearing never to be that stupid again. Then my dragon took her place next to me on the bed, sneering as she watched my despair. She swung and she scored and for the rest of the weekend retained her control over me. I quickly sank into a deep depression that immobilized me to the bed unable to do anything all weekend but cry and worry. Periodically I would unwrap my arm and compare it to my left arm to see if any of the swelling had subsided. I resorted to googling again, finding a video that described the proper way to wrap the arm in order to obtain the most benefit from it. We devised a makeshift handle from the ceiling to help keep my arm suspended when it became too heavy to hold up. By Monday morning we were exhausted, but had managed to reduce most of the swelling. Measuring the arm, it still remained a half inch bigger than my left arm.

I knew that I needed medical help with this. Each chemo, I speak with the onc about side effects that I am experiencing. I quickly explained what had happened over the weekend, displaying my right arm as evidence. Maybe he saw the angst in my eyes, but he didn't blow me off this time. Instead he made arrangements for me to be seen by a therapist especially skilled for lymphedema at which time I will be assessed and a plan will be instituted to keep my dragon and the lymphedema at bay.

Cancer: Lymphadema

Sometimes it seems like a new threat lurks around every corner. At times it seems as though I no sooner overcome one obstacle before I am running headlong into another one. There is always a dragon needing to be slain. There is too much cancer around me. It hangs like a dark cloud over the house. I sleep in it, work in it, eat in it, and exist in it. I keep thinking about a beach somewhere, with waves lapping at my feet, and a little umbrella drink with my name on it. The sun is always shining, but there is a cool breeze blowing gently against my face and the smell of the salt water teases my nostrils There is no cancer there, and my dragon is tethered to the same place I will have escaped from, so she is gratefully absent from my fantasy.

I need to find that place soon, and take a respite from this darkness around me. I need to shed this stench of cancer, even if only for a moment and drink in the fresh air. Two more chemos left to go and then what happens? I'm having some doubts about what takes place next.

The supposition is that the chemo will kill all or most of the cancer in my body. If any cancer remains, it will exist at a cellular level that will take time to develop. In my mind, that means that my breasts will be free of cancer, at least for now, so why cut them off now and add weeks of recovery to my life that has already been rudely interrupted by the cancer that hounds me? Why not wait until the cancer returns in the breasts before undergoing several more surgeries and their corresponding recovery times? Besides, maybe the cancer won't return to my breasts. Maybe the cancer will come through my bones, or my brain rather than my breasts. A woman in the cocktail lounge with me had started with breast cancer, but her cancer returned through her bones, not her breasts. I might be able to glean a couple of years of quasi-normalcy before I am forced to put my life on hold again.

I'm also questioning the radiation treatment that I am supposed to undergo because I've read that it can trigger the lymphedema as well. Radiation can cause scarring of tissue that serves to block the ability of draining protein rich fluids from the arm tissues. Will that aggravate things further, making the lymphedema worse? I'm not at all sure I am willing to risk that.

If I even scratch the arm I risk the possibility of infection that can create a septic condition that could be life threatening to me. I've already lost the entire summer putting my life on hold for cancer. I find myself unwilling to give it any more of my time right now. I want this roller coaster of emotions to stop for awhile. I realize that I cannot prevent the cancer from returning, and that I will forever be straddled with some aspects of this insidious disease, but there has to be a reprieve somewhere. There needs to be some opportunity for me to be me again. At some point, I will draw a line in the sand that will not be crossed. I just haven't decided when that will be yet.

There are lots of decisions yet to be made, and they are weighing me down. I just don't want to lose me and the person I have worked so hard to become.

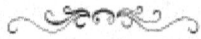

Cancer I did not give you the right,
To invade my body and take a bite.
This is my body and with all my might,
I will prevail with one hell of a fight.
To the cancer inside, I will battle and kill.
For that is my body's God given will.
To my cancer, these words I do send.
Your life is short and near the end.
(For Lucy & all those fighting cancer)
J Joens, 10/13/05

Cancer: God Incidence-
Wednesday, September 23, 2009

Today another chemo bracelet is removed leaving only one on my wrist. I wish that would symbolize the end of this journey, but I don't believe that this journey will end until I do, and then another journey will begin. Once you are diagnosed with cancer, your life changes forever. What you eat, how you live, and how you feel become forever meshed with the cancer cells that invade your body. Even if the chemo successfully kills the existing cancer, you spend the rest of your life fearing a recurrence. If it recurs, you are considered to be a stage 4, and the goal becomes prolonging life rather than curing it.

Visits to the cocktail lounge have become somewhat routine but never without their glitches. Since I am not allowed to drive myself to chemo because of the sedation, I depend on the assistance of friends to get me there. Yesterday was Sherry turn and she had no idea how long that day would become! For that matter, neither did I!

As usual, the first order of business is to jump on the office scale which confirms that the combination of steroids and insulin are turning me into a "sta-puff" marshmallow. From there a thirty minute wait in a sterile room devoid of magazines or reading material ushers in my audience with the onc. A short review of current symptoms and side effects and then I am on to the cocktail lounge and my companion, Ivy.

This time my interactions with the onc were more informative. I had been dealing with a new pain in my abdomen that was being treated as an infection. When the antibiotics ended and the pain remained, I feared the worst. The onc decided to put off a cat scan for an additional week because of my chronic kidney problems. He hoped the wait-and-see attitude would give the antibiotics a bit more time to work and work they did. By the time I visited the cocktail lounge, that pain had dissipated and I was greatly relieved.

The blood tests revealed that I have become anemic from the chemo, and that accounts for the extreme fatigue I have been experiencing. The onc explained that he would normally order a blood transfusion, but again, because of my fragile health, he chooses to wait and see if the number 9 drops to an 8 before he initiates such measures.

Because I have only one chemo left, I asked what would come next. I reminded him that the surgeon suggested a mastectomy. I have been weighing the possibility of postponing that procedure until if and when it surfaced again. I've already lost my entire summer to this insidious disease and I need a break. A mastectomy would mean at least one more surgery and recovery. Reconstruction would add an additional two or three surgeries that include an even more difficult recovery. If the cancer returns like they predict, and if it comes back in the breast, we can do it all then. But for now, I need some space from my dragon, and a chance to breathe some fresh cancer-free air. My onc reviewed the surgeon's records, and advised me that in normal circumstances he would concur with the advice of the surgeon, but in MY case (leave it to me to be different), going under the knife with my history of heart disease would be too risky, so he conceded that waiting would be his choice as well.

He asked if I had given thought to which radiation oncologist I would like to use for the upcoming series of radiation that will come next. I had, so I gave him the onc's name. I have some real fear about radiation because my research reveals that it may exacerbate the lymphedema in my right arm. I discussed the lymphedema in my last posting, so I won't elaborate on it here. As yet, I am still waiting for the compression sleeve to arrive that will adorn my right arm for the rest of my life. I will also be placed on a drug regime of herceptin for several years in the hope of preventing any recurrence. My cancer is fueled by estrogen, and the tamoxifen acts as a barrier between my body and it's access to that estrogen.

Once we had covered those issues, I was ushered into the cocktail lounge where the needle was inserted to my port, and Ivy was connected to the myriad of plastic tubing that hung from her. I get the benadryl first, which typically makes me tired. It's a small bag, so it empties quickly. Next is the taxotere which doesn't go well this time. My port doesn't usually work well because of a fibrin sheath that my body has grown around its opening causing blockage that delays the infusion process. This time the port was really misbehaving, and the infusion proceeded at a snail's pace. My normal 3 hour ritual turned into 5 once the taxotere was replaced by the Cytoxin, which is the last half of my treatment.

Poor Sherry had returned at the expected 3 hour interval only to spend an additional 2 hours patiently waiting for the end of the process so we could leave. She was more patient than I! As it turned out, we both believe it was a God-incidence, because just as they were *finally* dislodging the needle from my port her phone rang, and she was told that her mother had been taken to a hospital only 2 miles away from us. The delay afforded us an opportunity to detour to the hospital so that she could see her mom and gain some much needed reassurance that all would be alright. It never ceases to amaze me how God knows what's ahead and clears the way for it. To get a glimpse of

Cancer: God Incidence

that when it is happening is always exciting, and made the delay more acceptable. It was 8pm before we finally rolled into the driveway of my home.

Today I give myself my neulasta shot, which kicks my bone marrow into high gear. I have been bringing the shot home since my last chemo, and administering it here instead of driving all the way back to Davenport for a five minute injection. Wish I had thought of that sooner! Since administering it myself, it has come to light that much of my discomfort during chemo week is a result of this shot. Once given, it flattens me for several days with flu-like symptoms, extreme fatigue, fever, and muscle pains. There isn't much that can be done except to ride it out. Now that my blood glucose is stabilized, I seem to recover a couple of days sooner and that is a good thing! I decided to update my journal today because I know I won't have the strength tomorrow.

This past weekend 'Mas and I attended my 40th class reunion. It's hard to believe that it has been that long. I really needed a social event, and had a really good time. It was wonderful re-connecting with old friends and acquaintances. I have been mostly isolated with this cancer since the beginning. The constant trips to doctors and hospitals don't permit much time for socializing. Add to that the weeks that I am out of commission from the chemo and shots, and what little vertical time I have is spent trying to keep up with running our businesses. My onc keeps scolding me for taking on too much. I recognize that I need to cut back on some of my workload and start pacing myself, so I am planning to limit my involvement in the upcoming tax season. That always takes too much out of me when I am reasonably healthy. I can only imagine how things will go if I try to keep up that pace!

That brings me back to my understanding that a diagnosis of cancer is a life sentence. Life as you know it forever changes. There are dark days when I want my old life back, resenting this dragon that stalks me. But there are also good things that have come as a result of it. In an odd way, the cancer has forced the destruction of many of my protective walls that have served to keep people out most of my life. I don't know how I would get through this without the prayerful encouragement of friends and family. They have made a difference in fortifying my courage as well as my determination to slay this dragon if I can. Their friendship has comforted me with the knowledge that if I don't beat the odds, my life has still counted for something, and there will be people who will notice my absence. My life has had some purpose.

Without the push of cancer, I don't know if I would have overcome the damage of my childhood enough to open the doors of my heart. It's not easy accepting help from others when you are used to overcoming adversity alone. It's much easier to give than receive, which is a humbling experience, but the result is almost worth the consequences of cancer. I say almost because I still

99

would prefer a cancer-free life, but if I must endure this, it is so much better to do so with caring and encouraging friends. Whether I win, or whether I lose, I will have fought a good fight. During those positive times my dragon sulks in the shadows, knowing that the closeness of friends denies her a victory. She is a potent adversary, but I will slay her if I am able. Bring it on!

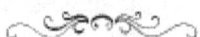

I have heard there are troubles of more than one kind.
Some come from ahead and some come from behind.
But I've bought a big bat. I'm all ready you see.
Now my troubles are going to have troubles with me!
~Dr. Seuss

Cancer: Cutting the Cord with Ivy-
Wednesday, October 14, 2009

Well, I finished my last chemo. The last bracelet has returned to the jewelry box as I breathe a sigh of relief. I realize that as this chapter of my journey closes, another one opens. Tonight I will take my last neulasta shot, and hopefully spend the last of what have been weeks confined to my bed.

Unfortunately, I will not get to that beach for awhile since I will be going right into radiation. I will meet with the new radiation oncologist next Monday at which time I will learn the schedule of the radiation process. As I understand it, the radiation is necessary to rid my body of any lingering cancer cells surrounding the area of the tumor that the chemo hasn't killed. Because I will be undergoing radiation every day for six weeks, we will attempt to start the process as soon as possible. I've been warned that the radiation will likely burn me, so this won't be a particularly pleasant experience either. I may also be subject to nausea, vomiting, fatigue, hair loss and anemia. Since I have already been dealing with all but the vomiting, I guess that won't pose any new issues for me.

As it turns out, I will also be receiving a PET scan on October 28. This scan will hopefully determine if the cancer had made its way into my lymph nodes to settle anywhere else in my body. If we don't find any signs of this, I can have the port removed. I think that the scan will provide some peace of mind, since the surgeon had told us that he stopped short of staging me as a IV because he couldn't tell me where it went when the cancer entered my lymph nodes. That has always left some question of whether the cancer had invaded any other organs before we found it.

The port has been a chronic and ongoing problem. I had asked for special prayers for the port yesterday because of my last experience with it. That day I was married to Ivy for more than 8 hours when the process is only supposed to take four hours! This week didn't show much promise either until I inadvertently shifted positions. I was stunned to look up and find the IV bag dripping like it was supposed to! Apparently the issue with the port is a positional one! All I had to do was shift onto my side and pull my legs up! Whooda thunk it?? I truly believe this is a God thing. For the past 5 months it never occurred to me to shift to my side. They have made me stand up, tilt right, tilt left, and lean forward, but never sit on my right hip! Such an easy solution to such a chronic problem! My God is such a smart guy! Not only did the port continue working the way it should, but I was out the door in four hours! Yippee!

I will still be visiting my onc every six months, and I will be taking a unique drug for several years in the hopes of preventing a recurrence which the doctors have also predicted as likely, if not probable. While I may not defeat this dragon over the long haul, I feel as though I have whipped her this time around. I won't know that for sure until we see the PET results, but I feel pretty confident at this point and she has gotten very quiet of late. Maybe she retired to that beach instead of me because I haven't noticed her lurking around here much lately.

There remain some serious challenges in our immediate future, and living with this dragon won't be easy, but we have made it this far, and God has promised that he won't bring us to it unless he plans to bring us through it. I've got a tight grip on that promise and I'm holding Him to it!

This seems like an appropriate time to thank everyone for their support, prayers and assistance throughout this ordeal thus far. I certainly couldn't have done it without each and every one of you! I will be eternally grateful for all you have done and I will always be available to return the favors whenever possible. I will never cease to be amazed by the importance of moral support when slaying a dragon like cancer. When I struggled through my weakest moments, there was always an angel who would enter the picture with a smile or a hug accompanied by a word of encouragement. Others quietly prayed, content to remain in the shadows lending strength and comfort through their prayers. Whatever your role was, I appreciated it! The battle isn't over yet, and I will still need your supportive prayers and encourage-ment as there are major challenges ahead that will certainly task us. But for now, this chapter closes with a victory that I share with each soul that earned it with me. I praise God for you!

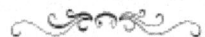

"Through humor, you can soften some of the worst blows that life delivers. And once you find laughter, no matter how painful your situation might be, you can survive it."

--Bill Cosby

Cancer: Radiating Hope-
Wednesday, October 21, 2009

I Had my visit with the new radiation onc. He seems like a nice guy. Even better, he doesn't mind answering questions! Too bad I didn't know which ones to ask yet! I'm finding that in this whirlwind called cancer, it's tough to stay one step ahead of the process with intelligent questions because you are so busy dealing with whatever is going on at the moment that there isn't time to foresee what's coming next!

As it turns out, the Trinity cancer center appears to be a very nice facility and the folks running the show seem very friendly. My radiation process will last every week day for seven weeks. The actual procedure will only take 30 minutes, so I will spend more time getting there and back than I will receiving treatment. At least this time I won't require a chauffeur, although I will probably get so bored driving back and forth that the company of a friend followed by shopping and errands will probably make for a welcome distraction on occasion. I realize that my dragon is always with me but she has become very quiet of late, and I don't allow anyone to smoke in my car. :^)

They can't actually start the radiation process until about three weeks following the end of my chemo, so we hope to get things kicked into gear by the first week in November. Meanwhile I will have a "markup" session next Tuesday wherein they tattoo the guiding marks on my body. When he said "tattoo" my eyebrows shot up. I'm needle phobic which has always inhibited me from getting a tattoo. (considering the four shots I gave myself a day now, that sounds laughable) I glanced over at my security blanket (read: 'Mas) and then asked if he could be with me during this precursory session. Due to the radiation present, the answer was "no". Bummer! How ironic that I am finally getting myself a tattoo and it won't even be a cute one!

It does occur to me that if for any reason this marking procedure desensitizes me to those tattoo needles, I might consider a very small dragon sporting a pink ribbon somewhere in an indiscreet location. Wouldn't that be a hoot? I've got a variety of things on my "bucket list", but getting a tattoo wasn't really among them. Of course, I am learning that I am never too old for changes, so why should this be any different?

I know that my dragon will accompany me on this little junket, even if my security blanket cannot. She doesn't have any problem with radiation, and she would love to hold my hand with her clammy, scaly fingers while she whispers frightening speculations in my ear. There are some things that I can depend on her for! She is quite the artist, and always good for drawing conclusions, most of which do NOT work in my favor!

Unlike my fear of the chemo, I have only one fear of the radiation (aside from those needles) and that would be the effect it might have on my lymphedema. Although getting the necessary arm sleeve has been one of the most frustrating experiences to date, I have finally opted to pay for it outright, eliminating the insurance equation due to the constant hassles. Thus it is on order, and by the time I start radiation I will be wearing it, which should help abate at least some of the negative effects. The new onc agreed that it would exacerbate the problem, but I was afraid to inquire as to how much. I've noticed that throughout this process thus far, I tend to avoid the questions that I don't want the answers to. I've always told others not to ask me a question unless they are prepared to hear my answer, so I guess I am living by my own decree. Well, at least I am consistent.

There are, not unexpectedly, a few side effects that I must brace for. (Gee, what a surprise!) Extreme fatigue...wow! now there's a surprise! Nausea..nothing new there. Hair loss...I think I have that one under control! Skin burns...okay, that's a new wrinkle. There are also some new rules. No deodorant...let me know if I start smelling like last week's garbage! NO HOT TUBBING! Ohhhh, a dagger to my heart! I have managed to devise a way of keeping my arm out of the water, but there is no way to avoid my armpit in the water. Obviously, this chapter of the experience isn't going to be a picnic either, but at least I won't be horizontal a week at a time! (I don't think! Unless that fatigue factor does me in!) The onc believes that this shouldn't present any issues for my heart although they have to penetrate the radiation all the way to my chest wall due to the depth necessary to find clean margins initially. I'm supposed to let them know if I experience shortness of breath. Now there's a yuck! With congestive heart failure, I've been experiencing that all along! Thus how would I know?

So at the end of my day, as the chemo chapter closed, the radiation chapter of my journey opened. Never a dull moment around here! My dragon is clapping her paws in anticipation. New fodder for emotional warfare, but this fodder is not as potent as the last. Her potential victories are losing their edge. She has one major event upcoming between the chemo and the radiation which is the PET scan. But that is a fight for another day. Today, I am just chilling in the knowledge that the chemo is finally over, and the radiation doesn't sound all that intimidating...YET! I am finally learning to take my battles as they come. I'm traveling lighter, as Max Lucado would say, knowing that wherever this journey leads me, I can look up and know that I am not going there alone.

One of these days

by FFH

One of these days I'm Gonna see the hand that took the nails for me

One of these days Gonna hold the key to the mansion built for me

One of these days Gonna walk the streets of gold that were paved for me

One of these days I'm gonna see my Savior face to face

One of these days

And one of these days I'm gonna talk with all the saints that have gone before

And in their sandals I will walk and we will sit along the shore

And I will learn all the things That I never knew before

All this and more

One of these days I'll finally be In a place where there's no more need

No more pain and no more grief no more foolish disbelief

And all the joy there will be when at last we finally see

One of these days

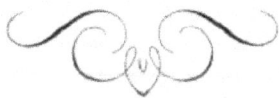

Cancer: The Cold Nose of a PET-
Friday, October 30, 2009

Today was supposed to be the BIG day. I finally had that PET scan that would confirm that the chemo had effectively eradicated the cancer that was invading my body. I was pumped up for good news as I stopped off at the imaging center to retrieve the report on my way to the radiation oncologist for my tattoos. The radiation was scheduled to begin in a week, and I was more than ready to move on to the next chapter of this journey. I ripped open the envelope as I walked through the exit door, excitedly reading the words as I hurried back to my car.

I say WAS as in the past tense. Things did not go as planned. The PET scan revealed "multiple, bilateral lesions" that had metastasized in my lungs. There were other words on the paper, but my eyes were riveted to the word "metastases". I read the paragraph again and again, convinced that I must not have read it correctly! Read it again, my brain kept screaming! As my brain tried to absorb the rest of the words. my eyes refused to move beyond the "m" word. I suddenly realized I had stopped breathing. Wow! Deja Vu! Breathe, Patti, breathe! Now we know where the cancer ended up.

There wasn't time to think at that moment. I steered my car out of the parking lot and across the road to the Cancer Center where my appointment with the radiation onc was waiting. On legs of rubber I walked the distance from my car into the building. With an expressionless face, I announced my arrival to the receptionist, who directed me into the waiting area. In short order, I was led back to an exam room by a smiling nurse who was obviously clueless to the news that was awaiting me, and unaware of the racing of my heart as I pushed the panic back before it choked me to death.

I waited what seemed like eons for the radiation onc to make his entrance. He wouldn't know that I already knew the bad news. I wondered if he was somewhere bracing himself for my anticipated reaction. As I positioned myself in the exam room, I opened the manila envelope that contained my fate, and read the words again, hoping that there was something I had missed that would make all of this go away. I took out my pen to jot down a couple of questions, and I underlined a couple of words that I was unsure of the meaning of. Next to the "m" word I penned the question, "Am I stage IV?"

While I waited, I retrieved the tape recorder from my purse. I knew that 'Mas would want to know everything the onc said and I didn't trust my chemo brain to retain it. The rad onc eventually appeared and seated himself on the stool in front of me. He didn't look me in the eye but rather busied himself opening and positioning my file on his lap. When he did glance up, he knew instantly that I knew and we both knew where this conversation was going. There would be no tattoos today. I had already swallowed the lump in my throat. I had already braced my feet as though I were standing in front of a moving bus, waiting for it to hit me. Next to the onc stood my dragon, wearing her best "I-told-you-so" sneer. Determined not to give her an inch, my eyes remained dry. The conversation that followed was as mechanically disconnected as a discussion about the weather would be at a funeral. We spoke enough to confirm that I understood what I had read correctly, that I was indeed Stage IV, and that the radiation was now a lower priority than the cancer that had revealed itself in my chest. I asked if we were now looking at prolonging life rather than curing cancer, and he indicated that this was probably the case. I asked if this meant more chemo, and he nodded his head affirmatively. It's back to the original onc for a further plan of action. This onc tried to be as upbeat as reality would allow, but that wasn't much. He wished me luck, offered to be available for any questions, and dismissed me.

In a fog I wandered back to the reception desk. As I walked past it, someone called my name. As I turned and looked, a nurse that I had met on Tuesday's visit threw her arms around my neck, wishing me luck. I muttered something about probably needing it, and resumed my path to the door. Once outside in the damp air, I realized how alone I felt, and reconsidered the wisdom in not bringing anyone with me. I reached for my cell phone and hit the speed dial to 'Mas. By the time I had finished talking to him, I had climbed into my car.

I realized that I wasn't alone. Looking upwards I verbally uttered, "okay, God. If this is your will for me, I'll do it. Just don't let go of me". I can't really explain the sense of peace that I experienced. I called my son and calmly explained what was happening. I called a few prayer warriors that should be notified. As though I was operating on auto pilot, I finished the one errand that I needed to complete, broke a nail in the process, and drove myself to the mall to get my nail fixed. Part of me wondered why I wasn't hysterical. Maybe I'm crazy? But I don't *feel* crazy! And I don't feel hysterical. I'm not sure WHAT I feel!

I decided that as long as I was at the mall to fix the nail I might as well get my nails done. 'Mas had called me to announce that he was too shook up to concentrate at work, so he was coming home. I wasn't ready to share tears yet. I called our friend Bobby and asked him to check in on 'Mas until I got there, secretly hoping that by the time I arrived, 'Mas would have worked through his own tears enough to not need to share any with me. I was grateful for the delay that the nails gave me. I just wasn't ready to start the wake yet, if you know what I mean.

Cancer: The Cold Nose of a PET

The trip home gave me more time to think. Ahh, here we go with the analysis! It occurred to me that maybe what was coming at the end of December was a God thing. Because of the upcoming circumstances of that, I was determined to get the port out. Getting the port out prompted the PET scan. If those events had not happened in that order, we would not know that my cancer had spread, and the need for more chemotherapy would have never surfaced. So is this God's way of bringing something to light that might have otherwise been overlooked? Following that logic, if God wanted it found, would that be because he knew that it had to be treated immediately if it is to be contained? A reasonable possibility in my book. I've seen God work that way before.

I narrowed my eyes as I averted them to my dragon seated next to the passenger door. "Not so fast, Dragon!" I hissed beneath my breath. "This fat lady hasn't sung yet!". As I write this, I still haven't decided if I'm privy to some spiritual knowledge that my conscious brain hasn't discovered yet, or if I am in a state of total denial, but as yet no tears have flowed, and I still am as calm as the proverbial cucumber. wow! What's up with that?? Maybe I am in a state of shock? Or maybe I instinctively saw this coming, so was already braced for it? Or MAYBE I'm just at peace because I know that whatever is happening, God is in control and I'm okay with that. I can't predict how I'll feel tomorrow.

'Mas and I will meet with the onc next Wednesday. By that time I will have done my research, and compiled my list of questions. I didn't ask initially, but now I want to know about a realistic prognosis. I want to know if I have time or not. My future direction will depend on some of these answers. The only thing I am sure of right now is that God is in control, and this will end however He wants it to end, and I will be alright with that.

My brother just called from Texas. He works in a medical nuclear lab. I read the report to him over the phone. His opinion is that I might have six months to a year, and his advice is that I get my house in order now. He suggests that since I will probably never see retirement, we should do what we want to do now while we still can, because lung cancer is going to be an arduous and painful way to leave this world. My dragon was listening to our conversation, and she is watching my face intently. While I believe that what my brother says may well be true, I'm not giving her the satisfaction of a reaction. I remain nonplussed by her presence. She may win this battle eventually, but it is not her time YET. That time is not her's to call. Only my God knows the time, and I have already started my preparations.

In his poem " The Prophet," Kahlil Gibron speaks of dying as he writes, "how shall I go in peace and without sorrow? Nay, not without a wound in the spirit shall I leave this city." But he also says, "Empty and dark shall I raise my lantern, and the Guardian of the night shall fill it with oil and he shall light it also." My Dragon will not win, no matter how my story ends. But she will likely never understand why. Too bad for her. I shall know why, and God will know why and that is all that will really matter.

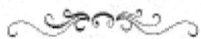

An individual doesn't get cancer, a family does

. ~ Terry Tempest Williams

Cancer: The Beginning of the End-

On Friday I wasn't sure whether I was in denial or shock, or simply had a peace that surpasses understanding. Today I'm pretty certain that it is the latter.

"Mas and I were ushered into the exam room where we took our seats and waited for the onc to make his appearance. When the onc finally took his seat on the stool, he looked at me sadly and announced that the news wasn't good. I looked him in the eye and said, "I know". He seemed taken aback by my pronouncement, so I explained how it was that I already knew about the lung cancer. His expression changed from sadness to relief. He explained that he had taken a couple of deep breaths and meditated a bit in preparation of giving me the news, so I was making his job easier for him. He asked if I wanted to see the PET scan and I apprised him that I had already seen it. Once again he seemed surprised. I described what I had seen on the scan, and reiterated my understanding that the brain, kidneys and bladder automatically light up due to the energy contained in them. I expressed my understanding that the bones that lit up had probably done so because of the neulasta shot, and I described the 6 or 7 various tumors that I believed I had seen representative of the cancer that had now overtaken my lungs. He commented that I knew as much about the PET scan as he did, and I responded with some vague comment about making it my business to know.

His reluctance to address my questions in the past was now a distant memory. I had his rapt attention as well as his apparent willingness to give me as much time as I required to understand what was happening to me now. He believed that a biopsy of the lungs was unnecessary under the circumstances, and he would prefer to spare me the discomfort of such a procedure. He was of the opinion that the cancer in my lungs had been there all along, and he assured me that even the stronger cocktail that I had passed over initially would not have cured me. What I have is incurable and further attempts to treat this cancer will be limited to slowing it down if possible. Since a cure is not in the cards, he will not subject me to the rigorous chemotherapy routine like I had just completed. Instead, he will provide me with a oral regiment of Herceptin.

Initially, my breast cancer was borderline HER+. I thought that it was determined to be HER2 negative. The good news is that because of the HER+, the administration of Herceptin might slow the cancer down, thus potentially buying me a little more time. The bad news is that when the cancer jumps to a different organ, the status of the HER is subject to change, and the cancer in my lungs may not be receptive to the Herceptin any longer, so the effort could be in vain. Only time will tell us the answer to that.

Since PET scans are expensive, he is opting for the simplest method of monitoring the lung cancer which is a chest x-ray. On the way home we stopped at Geneseo and took care of that. It is our hope that the cancer will adequately show up on the chest x-ray so that any growth can be detected and measured, which will tell us if the herceptin is working or not.

"So how much time do I realistically have?," I asked matter-of-factly. The average individual who has what I have will survive for one or two years. It's in God's hands now whether I last more or less time than that. He assured us that the cancer is in my blood stream and it *will* find other places to grow. He also informed us that the lungs harbor a much grimmer prognosis than if the cancer had found my bones instead. The sliver of good news is that the cancer is currently in my lungs and not in the lung lining. The lungs themselves have no nerve endings, so until the cancer finds another organ to invade, I will likely not experience any pain. I will develop a cough and I will have trouble breathing, but since the latter is a symptom of the congestive heart failure that I already have, I will probably not realize the symptoms at first. Another shred of good news was that the cancer has not found its way to my liver YET.

I will meet with the onc again next Tuesday, at which time he will begin the administration of the herceptin, and we will discuss what may or may not be visible on the x-ray. There isn't much else that he can do, so I will only have to return to the cocktail lounge every couple of months to be monitored. Eventually, when the cancer spreads further, the disease wracking my body will gradually debilitate me until my body physically gives up the good fight and I will die.

I told the onc that "Mas and I have some things I want to do while I am still able to do them, the first of which is driving to Arizona to see my daughter who I haven't seen in a couple of years. I still intend to find that beach! Lucky for us the PourHouse is a business that can go mobile with us, so we will be in a position to do some traveling.

I know that the end of my story won't be fun, and how I die is more than a little scary to me, but I know that my God is with me every step of the way and I will continue to run the race until I cannot run anymore. He surrounds me with loving friends and family that will provide an ample supply of comfort to me which gives me strength and reinforces my courage. I am okay

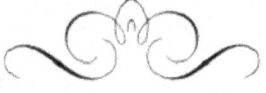

"Smiling Down"

by Pillar

You make it so hard on yourself
But there's nobody else
That could ever understand
The feelings that you felt
I could hear you think about
All the time I was around
If you could only see me now
I'm right here looking down
So next time that you feel like crying
Next time you don't feel like trying
Just remember I'll be right there smiling down on you
In the morning you don't feel like rising
Next time you feel like compromising
Just remember I'll be right there smiling down on you
I know you won't forget all the time we got to spend
Just because it's been a while doesn't mean that its the end
So right here and now I'll swear to you a vow
That I will always be with you whenever you feel down
Nothing ever will come between us
Now I'm holding on to the hand of Jesus
So next time that you feel like crying, Next time you don't feel like trying
Just remember I'll be right there Smiling down on you
In the morning you don't feel like rising,
Next time you feel like compromising
Just remember I'll be right there smiling down on you
I'll be right there looking down even when the shine don't shine
I'll be right there looking down all along the winter night
I'll be right there looking down with a smile on me face
I'll be right there with my arms open wide.
Right here on Jesus' side

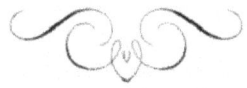

Cancer: One for the Gipper-
Tuesday, November 10, 2009

Author's Note: The Gipper was George Gipp who played on the 1916 - 1920 Notre Dame football teams under Coach Knute Rockne. On the evening of December 13, 1920 George Gipp died at the age of 25. In the 70's, President Reagan urges the Marines invading Granada to win it for the Gipper.

Today was another meeting with the onc to initiate the next phase of my treatment with the goal being to slow down the cancer since a cure is no longer an option. The chest x-ray reveals six cancer nodules in my lungs. The largest on the right lung is 2cm. The largest on the left lung is 1.8cm. They are very visible on the chest x-ray, which indicates that they are more advanced. I'm told that cancer doesn't show up on a chest x-ray until it is more advanced.

Today I met a new member of the staff by the name of Heather. Apparently she is some kind of nurse practitioner or something and she was the first person to see me and address any questions that I have. She was also the one that clarified that the 1-2 years life span estimate that I was given is contingent on my accepting more drugs to slow the cancer down. That came as a surprise to me. She confirmed that if I don't continue treatment, I will last a much shorter time. I don't know why that hadn't occurred to me until now, but it hadn't. When I finally saw the onc I ran that past him for confirmation. He made a face that put the truth to what I had heard as he said, "let's not go there."

Since the fish study had determined that I am HER2 negative, herceptin is not an option. I can't say I'm sorry about that because the research I did on that drug revealed a boat load of side effects. Instead, he described 3 different hormone drugs. To simplify an otherwise complicated explanation, I'll refer to them as small, medium and large. We are starting out with the smallest known to have the least side effects. It will become generic in 2010, thus making it more affordable sooner than the others. It's not very affordable right now! My 30 day supply rang the bell at $450! Thank God for copay!

I will go back on January 12 with another chest x-ray in tow to determine if the drug is working at all. If it slows any but not all of the six nodules he will consider it successful. He reminded me that this will only slow the cancer, not cure it. Yeah, I get it! If that drug fails to do the job, we'll move on to medium, and then to large respectively. The side effects to this drug are likely to be hot flashes and mood swings. Lovely! I thought I had finally gotten beyond those things seven years ago! I said, "Please tell me that I won't get PMS again!", but I'm remembering that the most stressful part of PMS was the mood swings! I thought about that t-shirt I saw that warned, "next mood swing in 6 seconds". Maybe I should get one of those so everyone has a fair warning in advance!

I asked the onc what would happen if none of the hormone drugs work. More chemo! Yuck! I looked at him with what would have been a furrowed brow if I had any brows! "We'll see," was my response. Chemo isn't his choice now because he wants me to have as much quality of life as possible. Well, we can agree on that one! Because of that, the port stays in indefinitely at this point. Speaking of the port, it has to be flushed out every six weeks. Since it had been nearly a month, the decision was made (not by me) to flush it today. It always hurts when they first poke that needle in. As usual, today was a day that the port decided not to cooperate, so the nurse had to get a longer needle. Did I mention that I am needle-phobic?? Today I got poked twice. I had never met this nurse before, so I had to wonder if the port was being that difficult or she was that inexperienced. I figured that the answer was probably a coin toss.

Next order of business was a warning by the onc that as soon as a tumor develops in another place, they might want to biopsy it and insure that the nature of my cancer (ER+PR+HER2-) hasn't changed. He won't biopsy the lungs because doing so would be too risky for me. It wasn't difficult for him to get across to me that a lung biopsy is not a pleasant experience, and since I am masochistically challenged, he'll get no argument from me!

My dragon keeps whispering that life expectancy estimation in my ear, giggling as she describes the drug side effects, knowing full well that I am without a choice here. If I want to live longer, AND I DO, refusing treatment is not an option. Until this was clarified, I had toyed with the idea of just stopping at this point. While there may certainly come a time when that will be precisely what I do, it won't be today.

Once Linda and I left the onc's office, I found the nearest SSI office in search of an application form. Amazingly, they don't provide blank applications anymore. The only way to apply for disability is to fill out an online form that asks more questions than the FBI! I explained that the nurses would fill out the papers for $20 which I thought would be money well spent. I was informed that they would have to come to the office to do that. Yeah, right! Like THAT'S going to happen! I left the SSI office annoyed, and I haven't even started the pills that cause the mood swings yet! This could get ugly!

We stopped for lunch across from Lowes and I remembered that I needed
something from Lowes, but for the life of me, had no idea what it could be.
How long does this chemo brain last?? I also remembered that I had received
a discount coupon for Kohls but I forgot that too! ARGH! No point in going
there either! I'm too cheap to buy anything without a potential 30% discount
coupon! My dragon slapped my forehead as though I could have had a V8!
Annoying yellow-eyed pain in the neck! Maybe the only good thing about
chemo brain is that I won't remember all those mood swings I will be having!
Is that a reasonable legal defense?

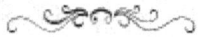

Cancer is not for sissies

~ Suzanne Somers

Cancer: Getting Opinionated-
Thursday, November 19, 2009

I guess if ever there were an appropriate time to seek a second opinion, it would be now. I received three phone calls within a 24 hour period regarding a breakthrough at Massachusetts General Hospital in Boston for lung cancer. Now oftentimes when God first speaks to me, I'm not paying attention, so he'll bring the subject around again. The second phone call got my attention enough to make me wonder if I was *supposed* to be paying attention. The third and last call drove me to their website to find out what all the hubbub was about for myself.

As it turns out, that breakthrough is for primary lung cancer. I don't have that. My lung cancer is metastatic lung cancer, meaning that it is the breast cancer relocated. I started to ponder why God would want me looking at Boston if he didn't have some kind of reason. In my experience, when I successfully follow through on one of God's plans, things just seem to fall into place like the pieces of a jigsaw puzzle. If it is actually my idea, things don't work out easily and I ending up smashing into a brick wall like a NASCAR smashing into the rail at 150 miles an hour.

Not to be dissuaded, I checked to see if this hospital and its doctors were in our insurance plan and they were! Now there's a switch! I then deferred to my old friend Google for the costs of getting to Boston. When I discovered getting there to be doable, I made an appointment with the Gillette Breast Cancer Center located at Massachusetts General for a second opinion. Because I believe that God is still in control, the appointment came through before the end of the year while the insurance remains in force. They may recommend the same treatments that my current onc is suggesting, but at least I will have tried to seek out the latest and the greatest possibilities for prolonging my life awhile longer.

Meanwhile I am still trying to find a middle road in my reactions to new pains. It's difficult not to panic when a pain turns up that hasn't been there previously and you can't explain how it got there, which is now the case for the left side of my neck. At my age, I can throw a muscle out of whack just sneezing, so I'm struggling not to let my imagination run away with me! On the other hand, what if this pain is significant? Should I have it checked? Part of me wants to run to the onc for some kind of reassurance. The rest of me figures that if it is still hurting by the time we head for Boston on December 8, they will investigate it like a heat seeking missile looking for its target and if it has any significance at all, we will know.

And what of my dragon, you ask? She's still lurking in the shadows, taking advantage of any opportunity to score points for intimidation. She loves instilling fear, and celebrates those new, unexplained pains for the confusion they cause me. While I convince myself that I am just overreacting, she whispers in my ear that the cancer has now spread to yet another location and even at a whisper, her voice can get loud!

I find myself less interested in work, and more interested in spending time around friends and family. Not a very practical approach to life if we plan to eat! My energy levels dissipate quickly so my projects seem to come together in short bursts which, for a workaholic like me, are something new. I tend to worry that I am getting lazy and that giving in to my fatigue is giving in to the cancer. I resist the urge to slow down, thinking that I'll get enough time for that when I am dead.

As each day passes, I wonder what the cancer in my body is doing. Is it multiplying like little rabbits? Is it stabilizing? Will I know if it takes a turn for the worse? How will I know? The questions are endless! My mind constantly churns them like butter. Like an unwelcome guest squatting in my guestroom, refusing to leave, this cancer has found a place in the depths of me. It has long since worn out its welcome, but it refuses to go. My dragon has staked out her claim to the bed across the hall, and she has made it clear that she doesn't plan to leave anytime soon.

That dragon is definitely wearing me down. My resignation is more apparent to me each day, which is one reason why I decided that a second opinion was in order. If there is any hope to hang onto, I need to find it soon. It's a long time to January 12 and the next onc visit, and thus a long time to wait for some hopeful information that the cancer is slowing down. Unlike the typical enemy in war, I cannot spy on her to see what she is up to. She has the advantage of surprise. Like a bogeyman lurking in the shadows she stalks me, and I peer carefully around each corner expecting her to jump out and shout, "BOO!"

Although I have been told where this is going, I haven't been privy to how I'll get there. That is the really scary part of the equation. Even if my dragon wins this battle, she needs to lose the war and I need to keep striving to insure that. I mustn't allow her to suck me into the undertow. I must not lose by default. As another survivor so aptly pointed out, there is no expiration date stamped on the bottom of my foot. I need to hold onto that.

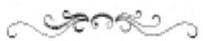

"Send Me A Song"
by Celtic Woman

Take the wave now and know that you're free,
Turn your back on the land face the sea,
Face the wind now so wild and so strong,
When you think of me,
Wave to me and send me a song.

Don't look back when you reach the new shore,
Don't forget what you're leaving me for,
Don't forget when you're missing me so,
Love must never hold,
Never hold tight but let go.

Oh the nights will be long,
When I'm not in your arms,
But I'll be in your song, That you sing to me, across the sea.
Somehow, someday, you will be far away,
So far from me and maybe one day,
I will follow you,
And all you do,
'Til then, send me a song.

When the sun sets the water on fire,
When the wind swells the sails of your hire,
Let the call of the bird on the wind,
Calm your sadness and loneliness,
And then start to sing to me,
I will sing to you,
If you promise to send me a song.

I walk by the shore and I hear,
Hear your song come so faint,
And so clear,
And I catch it, a breath on the wind,
And I smile and I sing you a song,
I will send you a song...

Afternoons with Ivy

I will sing you a song,
I will sing to you...
If you promise to send me a song.

Epilogue

While my race isn't over, and though my dragon has delivered a "technical knockout", I am hoping that the end of my story is awhile in coming. Nevertheless, this book has to reach some sort of conclusion. The announcement that my cancer will prove fatal seems to provide the pause that is needed for that purpose. My blog will continue, however, and if God is willing, perhaps a final chapter will be years in the offing. Whether or not that happens, I hope that my story, up to this point, can serve to encourage the next cancer survivor that crawls out from beneath that bus that hits her, and helps her to find the slivers of humor as well as the courage of conviction needed to fight the good fight. I also hope that my legacy can be one of a positive testimony to all that my God is a BIG God, and as such, capable of seeing us through whatever catastrophe awaits us. He remains in control. Remember that we all will die of something, and how we die is irrelevant when compared to how we live. As a wise person once said, "life is not measured by the breaths you take, but the moments that take your breath away." I have been blessed with so many moments that have done just that, and a plethora of friends to share them with. In that sense, I will die a rich woman.

Patti Gray-Pickering